Sarah Bayliss

Do Nourish

How to eat for resilience.

Published by
The Do Book Company 2025
Works in Progress Publishing Ltd
thedobook.co

Text © Sarah Bayliss 2025
Photography © Christian Banfield 2025
Illustration p39 © Patrick Filbee 2025

A CIP catalogue record for this book is
available from the British Library

ISBN 978-1-914168-38-3

To find out more about our company,
books and authors, please visit
thedobook.co or follow us **@dobookco**

5 per cent of our proceeds from the sale
of this book is given to The DO Lectures
to help it achieve its aim of making
positive change: **thedolectures.com**

Cover designed by James Victore
Book designed and set by Ratiotype

Printed and bound by OZGraf Print
on Munken, an FSC® certified paper

MIX
Paper | Supporting
responsible forestry
FSC® C163799

Disclaimer: Consult your doctor
before using this book if you have
a medical condition, are pregnant/
breastfeeding, take medication, are
a serious athlete, or have an eating
disorder. This information is for
education only, not medical advice.

10 9 8 7 6 5 4 3 2 1

Contents

The oak that withstands the storm
does not achieve its strength overnight,
nor through constant battling.
It grows slowly, drawing sustenance
from the earth, basking in the sun,
and swaying gently with the breeze.
So too must we build our resilience
— not through constant struggle,
but through patiently nurturing our
fundamental needs.

Eckhart Tolle

Prologue

Changing my relationship with food was my first step in becoming more resilient.

An early career in the fast-paced marketing world left me burned out, dealing with poor health and on the slippery path of neglecting my body's needs. It was tough being in an industry that expected me to work long hours, to exceed client expectations at every turn and had relentless social demands. I was living with disrupted routines, overdoing everything. My eating was erratic and I was always jumping from one fad diet to the next. The environment wasn't just draining my energy, it was robbing me of my health. I found myself feeling overwhelmed, unable to focus and think clearly and I struggled to make decisions. Sleepless nights, persistent digestive distress, including bloating and discomfort, low mood, self-doubt and loss of motivation became my normal. My appetite fluctuated wildly and ongoing mental and physical fatigue set in, resulting in persistent cravings for sugar and caffeine in an attempt to feel better and lift my mood. Even my hormones were affected, with noticeable changes to my menstrual cycle. I was worn out and knew I had to do something.

Eventually a move to Bristol and a change in job allowed me to re-evaluate my lifestyle choices. So, I began by making some simple changes: to my food and my sleep, and I set some boundaries around work and life. I couldn't believe that within a few months I had changed: my symptoms disappeared, my physiology improved and I had increased energy and focus. I felt more relaxed and far healthier.

This journey taught me that modern life often leads us to prioritise external pressures over our own needs. We develop coping mechanisms to manage the stress and the more we rely on them, the more ingrained they become. However, these self-protective behaviours are ultimately unsustainable. No matter how effective they might be in the short term, reality always catches up. Our bodies and minds can only endure so much before something inevitably gives way. The truth is, ignoring our fundamental needs and pushing ourselves beyond our limits will always have consequences, regardless of how well we think we are managing. Sooner or later, our health will force us to confront the reality we've been avoiding.

Many of the symptoms I experienced was my body telling me that something was wrong and at the time I wasn't listening. Being severely dyslexic, my strategy was to outwork and outperform everyone around me; thinking that if I achieved more, no one would suspect my perceived deficiencies. Maintaining that constant hustle, the people-pleasing and masking my struggles was utterly exhausting. It drained me of vital energy until my reserves were depleted. The saddest part was that I couldn't see how unhealthy these behaviours were.

Nutrition became my unexpected teacher. Changing my food helped me to listen to my body and intuition and to trust my gut (and look after it too). For the first time I could see how important it was to take care of myself.

Realising its power, I enrolled to study nutritional therapy to understand how nutrition and lifestyle behaviours impact health and performance. Having experienced the benefits first-hand and been empowered to help close friends and family, I became passionate about sharing this knowledge to help others achieve their own transformations.

My story is about slowing down, considering what really matters, learning to look after yourself. When you do, you have the energy to pursue what really matters. Your sense of purpose increases. You become more resilient.

This book is about how to build that kind of resilience. So many of us associate resilience with grit, determination and not giving up. And yes, working hard is part of the picture, but real, lasting resilience must be built from the ground up. We must understand the nutritional basics to give our bodies and brains the right resources to see and think clearly. To feel full and satisfied, so that ultimately you have the energy you need to sustain a busy lifestyle. But it's more than that. It's also strength and faster recovery; it means you have resources to bounce back quicker when things get tough.

And when you fuel from this place of resilience, magic happens. You have a far better understanding of what matters; you see a clear path forward. And with that clarity you have the power to focus and to take actions that change your circumstances for the better. You feel motivated, you start to believe that you can achieve your dreams and become the person you want to become.

You cannot do this from an undernourished body and mind. Trust me, I know.

My hope is that by reading this book, you'll discover a path to nourishing yourself in a joyful and satisfying way that fosters health and happiness; because that is what true resilience is all about.

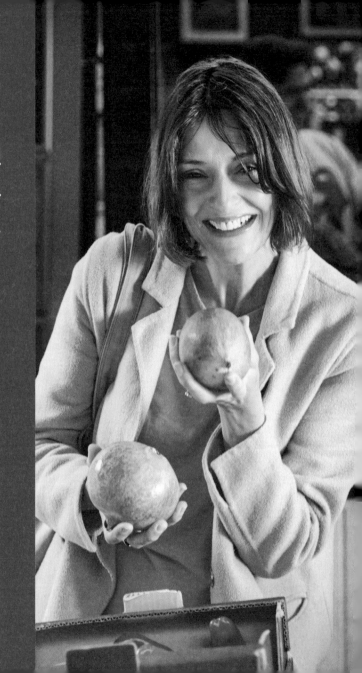

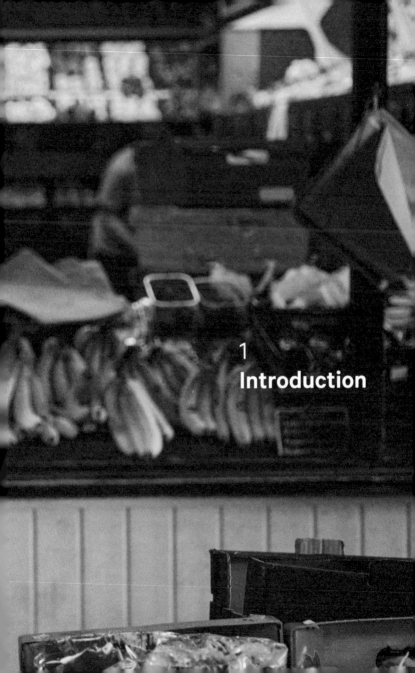

1
Introduction

> **What we do every day matters more than what we do once in a while.**
> Gretchen Rubin

At the heart of resilience lies metabolic health — it's the very foundation of how your body functions and thrives.

Metabolic health is the sum of many interconnected systems serving vital organs. It's your body's ability to convert food into energy efficiently, regulate blood sugar and manage hormones like insulin. When your metabolism is humming along, it provides your cells with good, efficient energy; the very fuel of resilience.

Think of it this way: when your cells receive poor energy, they can't carry out their functions properly. That's when disease risk increases, symptoms occur and your health takes a hit. But with good metabolic health, your cells are bathed in quality energy. This energy is the cornerstone of healthy ageing and robust resilience. It ensures a balanced and effective system in which organs and tissues are sufficiently fuelled to work seamlessly together, supporting not just your life, but your ability to bounce back, to push forward and to thrive.

In essence, metabolic health is about building a resilient body from the inside out; one that can weather storms, recover quickly and give you the vitality to pursue what truly matters.

In turn, how you live your life, the food you choose to eat, how you think about your food, your lifestyle and your life exposures control your metabolic resilience.

When it comes to your metabolic health there are seven key factors that influence how well it works:

— **Nutrition**
— **Sleep**
— **Stress**
— **Gut health and your microbiome**
— **Environmental toxins**
— **Movement**
— **Natural light and dark**

This book focuses primarily on one of these factors: nutrition.

I believe nutrition stands out as the most important and influential factor impacting health resilience. Food holds immense power — it serves as a tool that we can use to change our health and vitality, as well as how we think and feel.

Do Nourish will break down the basics of healthy eating to help you fit it into your life seamlessly. This project is my dedicated effort to make nutrition easy to grasp, so that you can enjoy living better.

A way of life

We are now more aware than ever that what we eat directly affects our health — how well our cells and organs function is based on the food choices we make.

My biggest aims with this book are to change how you think about your food by helping you understand nutritional basics and to give you an empowered understanding of what to eat. While the science might seem complex, the answers are straightforward. By the end you'll have a customised plan, feel motivated and know that this is a way of life, not a short-term way of eating.

There are two key factors that will determine your success in nourishing yourself well. Firstly, there are the consistent actions you take: small, simple steps in adjusting your food choices that I will guide you through. But the second factor is just as crucial — it's your underlying mindset and emotional relationship with making these changes. In other words, believing in what you are doing and understanding the 'why you are doing this' in order to make these nutritional shifts. Because at the end of the day, you are what you think. Your mindset matters.

My role is to be your partner on both fronts: I'll give you the practical 'what to do', but I'll also cultivate the 'why' through helping you to understand a little of the science and rationale behind the changes you're making. Having this deeper level of context will help you to truly believe in the 'why', which provides both motivational fuel and enhances your ability to achieve better physiological results. Science has shown us that what we believe is a powerful influencer on our physiology.

A bit about me

I am a registered nutritional therapist living in Bristol with a private practice helping clients improve their health in order to achieve a higher quality of life. I do this through personalised, functional nutrition with a focus on metabolic health, energy and stress management.

Functional nutrition takes a whole-body approach to optimal health by examining how the body's interconnected systems influence each other. Through that, I identify risk factors and/or find underlying imbalances driving a client's symptoms rather than just treating isolated symptoms or surface-level issues. Together we create a personalised nutrition and lifestyle plan, one that blends seamlessly into their life and daily rhythms. It's about creating something sustainable and achievable. My role is to meet the client where they are at, understand their vision and then guide and motivate them every step of the way. I help them feel inspired and empowered with knowledge about how their choices influence their mind and body. It's never about judgement, it's about building their customised roadmap for better overall health.

Imagine yourself as a strong tree. Your branches represent the various systems of your body: digestion, immunity, cardiovascular health and more. Just as a tree needs sturdy, nourished roots hidden underground to thrive, your overall health depends on a solid foundation. This foundation is built upon five pillars: what you eat, how you sleep, how you move, how you manage stress, and the strength of your relationships. By carefully tending to these 'roots', you establish a robust base for your health, allowing all your systems to flourish like vibrant branches on a healthy tree. Your body is an amazing integrated system, and creating true heath means nurturing the roots that shape you.

I have had the honour of working with many clients to help improve their long-term health. How do I know this process works? Because of my own experiences. I believe I can approach their need for change with empathy, coupled with the motivating factors of having derived the benefits of these lifestyle changes myself.

My approach in clinic is about making small sustainable changes that don't have to be a struggle. Small shifts can have a profound impact on your wellbeing. This is what happened to me and what many of my clients have expressed — they often tell me that my approach doesn't feel difficult. And that's precisely the goal: to guide people through an effortless transition towards a healthier, more balanced lifestyle. By understanding personal difficulties and finding workable solutions that fit into a client's life with minimal disruption, I can create practical results and the motivation to continue along this path.

I can honestly say I have never felt this great. Now I know what that feels like, I feel privileged that I can share this knowledge with others and witness their results. In writing this book I hope to be able to help more people. If, by reading it, you find a healthier path, then my work is done. Just like in my clinic, we are a team working together to live better.

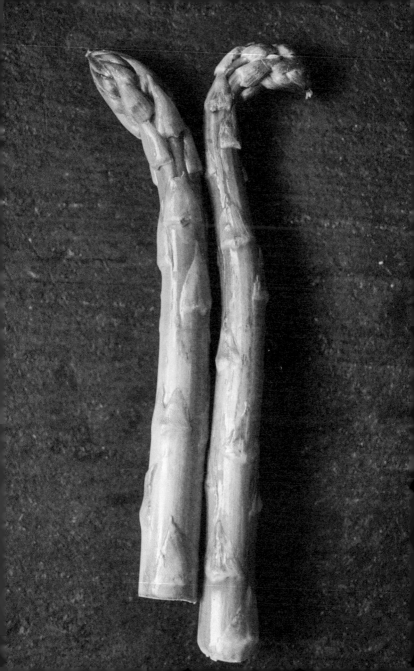

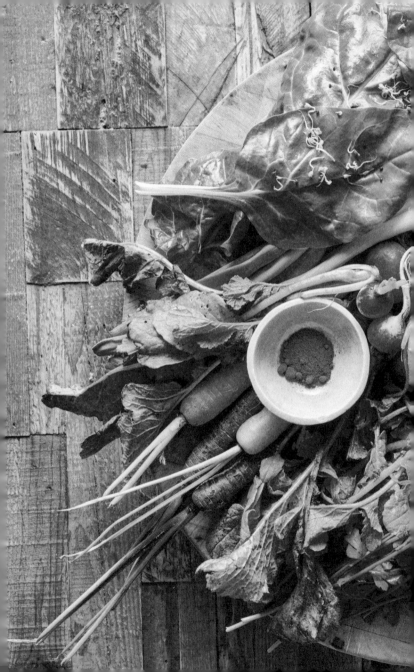

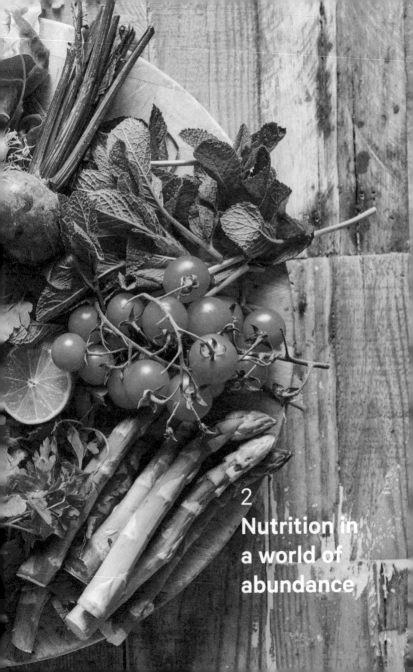

2
**Nutrition in
a world of
abundance**

If you don't feel you have time for health, how the heck are you gonna have time for sickness?

Dr Gabrielle Lyon

Staying healthy can sometimes feel like an uphill battle.

The wellness world bombards us with so much noise that it's tough to separate fact from fad. Contradictory advice, strict regimens, endless lists of must-haves to become our 'best selves'—it can feel overwhelming. Even as we gain more knowledge, new nutritional studies can just muddy the waters.

But it's not just the information overload making health a challenge. Our modern lives are stacked against us. Many of us are chronically stressed, running on empty from lack of sleep and overwork, never getting a chance to truly recharge. Making unhealthy choices has become too easy. We chase quick fixes like caffeine and dopamine hits to cope with the daily grind. It's a persistent battle between living for the moment and investing in our future selves.

Does this sound familiar? So many of my clients feel this way.

The current landscape may leave you feeling pretty gloomy, but there is hope. There is a different narrative and a more balanced way to live in the world. But first, I believe it's important for you to understand what you're up against.

Processed and ultra-processed foods

Historically, food processing arose from the need to cook foods in a way that made them safer and more digestible, as well as to preserve them and extend their life using methods such as salting and fermentation.

The industrial revolution marked a significant shift in the evolution of food processing. Innovations like tinned food and pasteurisation were introduced, which not only improved preservation, but created convenient, ready-to-eat options.

Processing has undergone a dramatic transformation since then. While it once focused on adding basic ingredients like salt, sugar and unhealthy fats to produce these convenient foods with lower nutritional value, food processing has progressed to the production of ultra-processed foods (UPFs). In addition to the added sugars and unhealthy fats, these UPFs contain a multitude of additives, drug-like chemicals, refined ingredients and artificial flavours, all of which raise significant health concerns.

In a lecture at the University of California, Dr Robert Lustig, the American paediatric endocrinologist, described UPFs as: 'not just different from whole foods; they are fundamentally different in the way they affect our brains and bodies. They are engineered to be hyper-palatable, addictive and calorie-dense, leading to overconsumption and negative health consequences.'

The challenge we face is that our shops and supermarkets are flooded with these highly processed foods and refined carbohydrates that lack nutrition and fibre. UPFs are often packaged in bright, appealing ways that make them look harmless. Many of them are even marketed as being 'healthy', and, of course, they taste great. However, beneath the attractive packaging and delicious flavours lie ingredients

NUTRITION IN A WORLD OF ABUNDANCE

21

that are designed to disrupt our metabolism. Dr Georgia Ede, a Harved-trained psychiatrist specialising in nutritional and metabolic psychiatry, said of UPFs: 'These products may look innocent and delicious, but concealed within their pleasing packaging are ingredients with the power to destroy your good mental and physical health.'

Recent research has suggested that ultra-processed foods are as addictive as smoking, based on their effects on the brain's reward system. They fool the brain into experiencing heightened levels of pleasure and have the potential to trigger compulsive consumption. And frankly, our bodies were never designed to cope with their levels of toxicity.

An over-reliance on processed food may also have eroded some of our natural understanding of nutrition and the origins of our food. When we cook from scratch, it instils an appreciation for ingredients, quality and the effort involved. I vividly recall my grandma's cakes. Baking with her, I knew precisely what ingredients were used and the love she poured into making then. We ate them on special occasions and savoured every mouthful.

Some processed foods can be part of a healthy eating plan and are convenient and helpful during busy times, for example frozen fruit and vegetables, high-quality protein powders, tinned beans, plain Greek yoghurt, tinned sustainable wild fish and condiments with no added sugar, oils, chemicals or preservatives. However, ultra-processed foods, which include added preservatives, colourings, flavourings and emulsifiers, go beyond mere convenience and are much more damaging. When differentiating between processed and ultra-processed, a good rule of thumb is to look at the ingredients list. If it has five items or fewer, it's likely just to be convenient. If it has more than five ingredients and contains items you don't recognise, then it's probably ultra-processed. If choosing convenient foods, just bear in mind that these foods can still have added sugar, salt and oils, and if they do you want to avoid them. Eating for resilience is about looking at labels, ensuring that what you buy is minimally processed, without added salt, sugar and oils, and buying organic ingredients where possible.

Provenance matters

Conventional farming practices rely on synthetic fertilisers and pesticides, which degrade soil health and affect crops and animals because livestock consume food loaded with chemicals. These practices lead to less nutritious food and have potentially harmful effects on animal and human health. Organic farming offers an alternative by restricting the use of synthetic fertilisers and pesticides, resulting in fewer toxic chemicals in circulation and food that is more nutrient-dense. However, while organic meat and dairy comes from animals not fed by synthetic pesticides, these animals may still consume an unnatural diet. The best thing to look for is organic and grass-fed meat and dairy. Regenerative farming goes one step further, focusing on soil health and biodiversity. This method avoids synthetic chemicals and employs practices that enrich soil nutrients and microbial life. In regenerative systems, animals graze freely, naturally fertilising the land and improving soil quality. For the best quality food consider buying local produce, ideally organic and regeneratively grown, as much as possible. You may have to pay more for these foods up front, but they will help you in the long run.

Hidden hunger

The Western world boasts an abundance of food, but nutrient deficiencies persist and the gap between what our bodies need and what we feed them continues to grow. This results in a growing chance of long-standing health problems and a higher risk of chronic disease.

Our modern lifestyle throws so many factors at us that contribute to a decline in our overall health. When you step back, it's easy to see how all these different elements are contributing to the broader health challenges plaguing society today. It's a complex, multifaceted situation without any single root cause. These factors include:

1. **Changing eating habits:** the way we buy, prepare and eat food has drastically changed.

2. **A rise in ultra-processed foods:** highly palatable, rich in calories but low in nutrition.

3. **Decline in food quality:** the quality of our soil is diminishing and our food travels further — both affect our food's nutrient levels.

4. **Toxins everywhere:** our exposure to environmental chemicals is growing and is often linked to health issues like obesity and metabolic disorders.

5. **Mounting stress:** our lives are becoming increasingly stressful, with constant data bombardment, overscheduled days and 24-hour news cycles triggering stress reactions from morning to night.

6. **Sleep struggles:** blurred day and night boundaries are causing erratic schedules and overstimulation, which affect sleep quality and quantity.

7. **Rising nutrient demands:** our bodies require a higher level of nutrients to cope with daily demands placed on them and help eliminate toxins.

8. **Lack of nutrition:** less than 10 per cent of most Western populations consume enough whole fruits and dietary fibre.

In short, we are not getting what we need. Our bodies don't operate in isolated bubbles. We're not a closed system. As I said at the start, our environment, social interactions, diets, gut bacteria, stress levels — all these external factors directly impact how efficiently our bodies metabolise and extract energy from food. Metabolic health is shaped by our whole lifestyle and surroundings, not just nutrition alone.

Food is one part of the equation for positive life changes. Changing nutritional habits must go hand-in-hand with making mindful decisions about your overall environment and lifestyle, such as taking breaks from screens and ensuring a good night's sleep. These restorative practices will allow clarity to emerge so you can begin to make more intentional choices about what you eat.

How to use this book

Changing our habits can be tough because most of our daily decisions happen on autopilot — they are driven by our subconscious beliefs and ingrained patterns. Our conscious mind is only active for about 5 per cent of the day. To change any habit, we need to start with awareness — slowing down to notice and recognise the choices we're making. Without that awareness, real change is nearly impossible.

Since most of our food decisions happen in the unconscious mind, we need to bring about change slowly and work with your existing eating patterns. Let's start with some good news: you're already eating food, so you don't have to build an entirely new habit from scratch. You just need to adapt how and what you're eating. That's a much easier win and gives you a great head start.

Clients often say to me, 'Just tell me what to eat. Give me a 7-day meal plan to follow so I don't have to think about it.' On paper, that sounds great, but in reality, it requires a lot of mental effort: reading recipes, buying new ingredients, changing your grocery shopping, following the steps. It can be a lot of change at once.

Everyone loves recipes, and my clients are usually happy to try new ones on weekends or when they have more time. But following a rigid 7-day meal plan from the start is tough; it taxes your working memory (your brain's short-term information processing system, which helps you manage and carry out immediate tasks). When you are juggling multiple tasks in your everyday life on top of new recipes, ingredients and new cooking styles you can quickly become overwhelmed. And it becomes even more challenging if you are cooking for an entire family.

In my clinic, I often don't provide recipes until the second or third consultation because what I've found is that when clients understand what they need to eat for optimal function and can adapt parts of their current routine, they have much greater success.

The approach in this book aims to be uncomplicated. I have designed a 6-week plan in which, each week, you'll focus on one 'pillar of nourishment' and address or enhance how you're currently eating by adapting just one part of your plate. The idea is that you should hopefully be able to align the steps outlined with your existing habits by making one change at a time. Over time, these small changes will build up to create a balanced, nourishing meal — no matter where you're starting from.

I've designed it as a 6-week plan, but you can accelerate through multiple weeks if you're ready for faster change or take it much slower if you need more time to adjust. I'd recommend taking it one week at a time and see how you feel before moving forward. If you've found a particular week's change difficult, then keep that as your sole challenge until it has become a natural part of your routine, then move on to the next week's pillar. The key is to progress at your own pace. It might take you a full year to make every single change and that's okay — you're still working towards enhanced health and wellbeing.

This approach is designed to give you what you need, with the hope that, over time, as you eat more of what your body needs, you'll have increased the good stuff to the point where the bad stuff slowly disappears.

I invite you to refer to chapter 11 at any point along the six weeks. This chapter is designed to help you bring more flavour and excitement to your food and will prove helpful if you're feeling stuck or uninspired about what to cook.

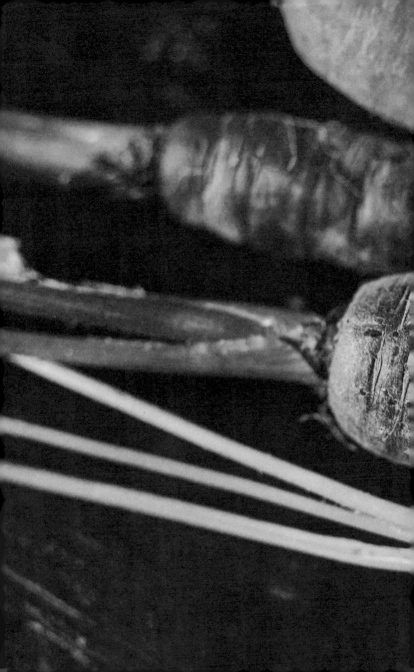

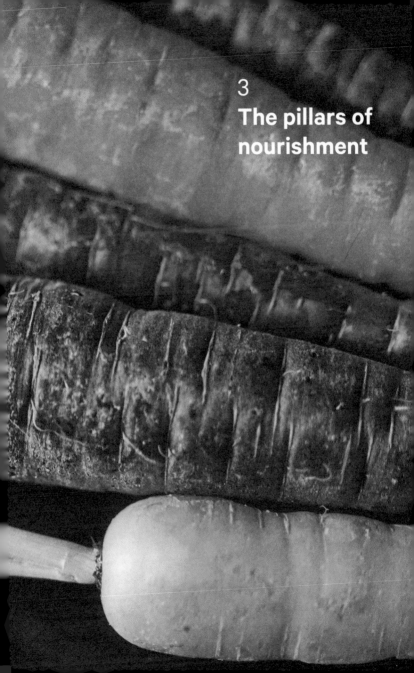

3
**The pillars of
nourishment**

Pleasure is short-lived.
Happiness is long-lived.

Professor Robert Lustig

Many people think nutrition is just about eating delicious food and that when life gets stressful, having a tasty treat can make us feel better; even if this is short-lived.

Real nutrition is about more than delicious food. When we eat nutritious food it fills our 'resilience bucket'. It gives us the ability to think clearly, make conscious decisions, handle whatever life throws at us and recover more quickly. But many people don't realise the connection between what they eat and how resilient they feel mentally and physically. Just as nutritious foods can energise our minds and bodies, unhealthy eating habits can drain us over time.

In this chapter, I want to share with you the basic foundations of nutritional resilience to give you the context of what nutrients the body needs but cannot make, and to steer you away from the idea that food is only fuel. I call these foundations the 'pillars of nourishment'.

Food is information. It's a message to the body that influences your biology and how your cells function. Your body is a complex network of systems and processes; you have a microbiome, an immune system, hormones, neurotransmitters and messenger molecules, all of which are influenced not just by the calorie intake, but by the informational qualities of the food you are eating. The food you choose has a profound effect on everything in your body and that effect can be dramatically different depending on its nutritional make-up. Understanding this concept will transform your perspective and the choices you make.

Your goal is to start eating in alignment with your body's physiological needs. By prioritising the nutrients that are essential for your body, you will feel full and satisfied, diminish cravings and increase energy and functioning. Remember, the perfect nutrition plan is the one that works for you and meets your physiological requirements. It must also be one that you enjoy.

To begin, we must briefly talk about how your body makes and uses energy. Your daily fluctuations in blood sugar and insulin levels serve as vital health markers, greatly influencing how you use or store energy. They play a key role in determining your overall resilience and susceptibility to disease.

Introducing insulin

I am going to get a little sciency here, but this section is super important — the information will help you understand why your food choices matter so much.

Glucose is a simple sugar that serves as your primary source of energy for your body. It is derived from many foods, including carbohydrates, fruits, vegetables and grains. When you eat these foods they are broken down during digestion and the glucose is released into your bloodstream. This glucose now circulates in your blood as blood sugar, ready to be used to fuel your cells and organs. Glucose is a critical energy source for many cells.

Insulin is a hormone that is produced in the pancreas and circulates in the blood, influencing various tissues in the body. Its main role is to get the glucose that is now in your blood into cells to be used for energy or stored away. It acts like a key, unlocking cell doors so that glucose can get inside. Every cell has insulin receptors to receive this fuel source.

Insulin tightly controls the amount of glucose in your bloodstream at any given time (only about one teaspoon's worth). Too much glucose is toxic to cells and your brain, as it can bind to proteins, fats and DNA through a process called glycation, impairing their normal function.

Once the glucose is inside the cell, the mitochondria — known as the powerhouses of cells — take the glucose and convert it into the energy currency of your body, known as ATP (adenosine triphosphate), so the cell can use the energy to do its many jobs. Every cell in the body has mitochondria to fuel its function; some cells have more, some have less, depending on the amount of work they need to do and their energy requirements. When the mitochondria are fuelled with appropriate nutrients, they can function well and produce ATP efficiently.

Carbohydrates, particularly simple and refined ones (you'll learn what these are in chapter 8) contain the most glucose and have the biggest impact on blood sugar levels. Sugar and processed foods also fall into this category. When you eat too much of these foods, your blood sugar level rises too quickly. To compensate, your body pumps out an excessive amount of insulin (above normal levels) to try to bring your blood sugar levels back down. This overproduction then causes your blood sugar to plummet just as quickly as it spiked.

Your brain perceives these dramatic blood sugar drops as an emergency. It responds by releasing various hormones to prevent your glucose from falling too low. Unfortunately, these hormones disrupt your body's energy system and resilience. They promote fat storage, impair fat burning, impair appetite control and activate your stress response.

These hormones are so powerful, they put you into 'fight or flight' mode — the stress system that can affect your whole body. Your heart may race, your blood pressure may rise, you can feel anxious, irritable, shaky, start to sweat and can lose concentration and focus. Ultimately, your resilience is in jeopardy. You are in survival mode, likely not thinking clearly, your cognitive function is diminished, and your brain is telling you to seek sugar and/or caffeine to refocus your mind. This is probably driving poor choices that only exasperate the situation. You can end up in a vicious cycle. Research has now also linked these blood sugar dips with anxiety and low mood.

Depending on how you are eating and what you are eating these blood sugar episodes can happen several times a day and into night and the more carbohydrates and processed foods you eat, the more extreme they will be. These steep ups and downs create hormonal havoc, continually throwing your energy system out of balance.

Simultaneously, while your blood sugar is riding this roller coaster, your mitochondria are being overwhelmed. They become overloaded with erratic fuel delivery, under resourced and stressed. Over time, this onslaught of improper fuelling can actually damage your mitochondria, making them less efficient.

The blood sugar roller coaster

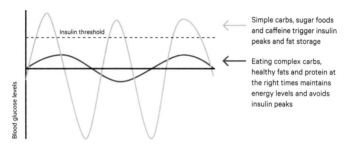

Blood glucose levels

Insulin threshold

Simple carbs, sugar foods and caffeine trigger insulin peaks and fat storage

Eating complex carbs, healthy fats and protein at the right times maintains energy levels and avoids insulin peaks

If this dysfunctional cycle continues over months and years, insulin resistance can develop. Cells become overwhelmed by the excessive insulin surges and stop responding appropriately. This triggers a vicious cycle of persistently elevated blood glucose and insulin levels. Your energy production systems remain disrupted, as glucose can't properly enter cells. The surplus gets shunted into fat storage instead, contributing to unhealthy visceral fat accumulation around your organs.

You eventually end up with a triple whammy:

— Persistently high, toxic glucose levels in your blood

— Chronically elevated, pro-inflammatory insulin

— Overwhelmed, dysfunctional mitochondria struggling to meet energy demands

With this systemic dysfunction, cells and organs become depleted of the quality energy needed to carry out their roles properly. This metabolic dysfunction and mitochondrial impairment opens the door to chronic diseases like type 2 diabetes, cardiovascular disease, polycystic ovarian syndrome (PCOS) and Alzheimer's, as well as impacting your day-to-day resilience.

Nutrition plays a pivotal role in keeping insulin balanced and properly fuelling your mitochondria. We need controlled insulin release, not excessive spikes. And your mitochondria need quality nutrient sources.

Just a note on alcohol — research suggests that alcohol is not metabolised by insulin. However, the body will prioritise alcohol metabolism, which can disrupt insulin's normal function in regulating blood glucose levels and can lead to elevated blood sugar and liver overload. Alcohol can reduce sleep quality and negatively impact our food choices. Heavy use damages the liver, disrupts the gut and increases inflammation. If you drink, choose organic, where possible, and avoid excess simple sugars like mixers.

Give your body the foods it cannot make

Your body has the remarkable ability to produce all the glucose it needs through various processes, ensuring a constant energy supply; however, it lacks the ability to synthesise essential nutrients that are crucial for maintaining optimal health.

Let's start with the big three macronutrients. These are the nutrients your body needs in large amounts. Only two of them are considered essential:

— **Carbohydrates**
— **Proteins** (known as essential amino acids)
— **Fats** (known as essential fatty acids)

In addition, there are essential components your body needs called micronutrients, which include vitamins and minerals. You need these in small amounts, but they are very important and help your body run smoothly.

Your mitochondria cannot produce energy without essential nutrients, so throughout this book, I will emphasise the importance of prioritising proteins, key fats and plant foods to meet your needs. As you work through the book, you'll begin to pay attention to your meals' nutritional composition and create a 'balanced plate' that supports your body's essential functions while helping keep insulin levels low.

When you provide consistent, high-quality energy sources, every single cell receives the nutrients it needs to function optimally. You are in balance, feel powerful and energised and your brain works at full capacity. When you are truly nourished, that's when happiness freely flows — at least I think it does!

So, let's meet the five pillars of nourishment: protein, healthy fats, non-starchy vegetables, complex carbs and polyphenols. At mealtimes, your ideal plate will contain each of the five.

I'll be explaining what each one is in detail, but for now, here is an overview, and what you'll be working towards at all main meals.

Protein

— ¼ of your plate or 1–2 palm-sized portions

Function: Protein (known as amino acids) are the building blocks of your body, keeping you strong and healthy. It builds and repairs tissues (such as bones), muscles (especially crucial as we age!), and keeps you feeling fuller for longer. But that's not all. Protein also plays a role in your metabolism, weight management, immunity, brain function and even helps with detoxification. Not getting enough protein can lead to cravings and increase your risk of developing bone problems, such as osteopenia and osteoporosis.

Healthy fats

— *1–2 portions per meal (1 portion is the size of 2 of your thumbs)*

Function: Healthy fats are an energy source to fuel cells, but they are also more than that. They make up your cell membranes, the structural layer around cells, which are critical for all aspects of health and control everything that goes into the cell to ensure it functions. These fats help support a healthy heart and cardiovascular system, a sharp brain, a strong immune system and help stabilise energy levels. Plus, they even act as antioxidants, helping your body fight free radicals.

Non-starchy veg

— *½ of your plate*

Function: Packed with rich fibre to look after your gut health and loaded with essential vitamin and minerals, non-starchy veg are vital for your immune function, brain function, energy production and many other processes in the body. They are gold dust for your metabolism and help ensure all cells run smoothly.

Complex carbs

— *approximately 1 cupped handful*

Function: An energy source to fuel cells. Carbohydrates have the biggest impact on insulin and blood sugar.

Polyphenols

— to add flavour to your food

Function: A group of plant compounds that has health benefits. They are found in large amounts in fruits and vegetables, as well as spices and herbs. They possess well-researched antioxidant properties that have been shown to inhibit inflammation, support metabolic health and gut health, protect the brain and reduce the risk of systemic disease.

What does a balanced plate look like?

It's important to note that these are guidelines. You are unique and your plate may require adjustments depending on your activity level and health status — so know that it is flexible. For now, just make a note of the balance and as you work through each chapter you will begin to build your ideal plate.

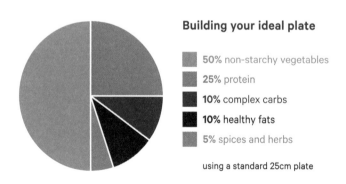

Building your ideal plate

50% non-starchy vegetables

25% protein

10% complex carbs

10% healthy fats

5% spices and herbs

using a standard 25cm plate

Measuring your portions using your hands as a guide

Protein
1-2 palm-sized portions

Healthy fats
2 thumb-sized portions

Non-starchy veg
2 handfuls

Complex carbs
1 cupped handful

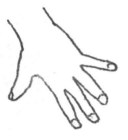

A palm sized portion

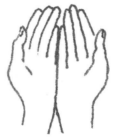

Two handfuls

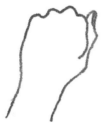

A cupped handful

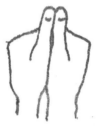

Two thumbs

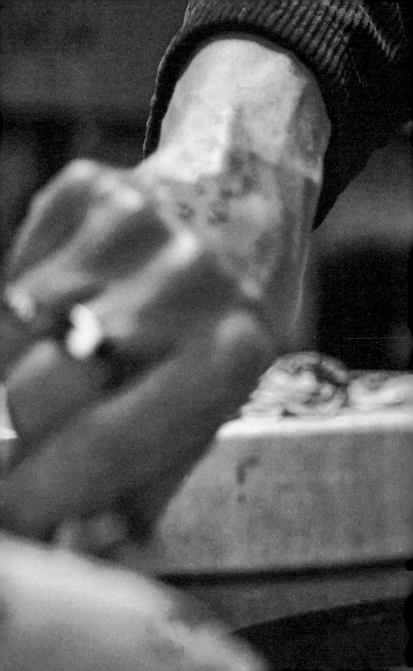

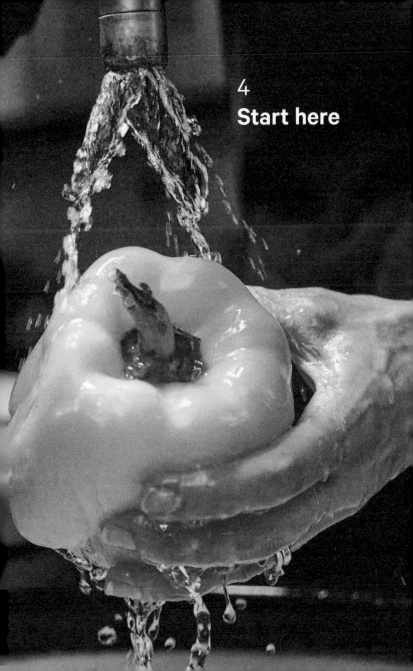

Making better decisions starts with having more self-awareness about your current eating habits and behaviours. Often, there's a disconnect between what we think we're doing versus what we're actually doing.

This chapter is about starting with complete honesty and zero self-judgement. By getting clear on your habits right now, you can make a realistic plan for the nutrition changes you need to make. Remember, sustainable changes take time. This process may take a few weeks or months depending on your current habits. Being totally upfront with yourself is key to successful behaviour change. In my clinic, when clients share their real food diaries, they're often surprised by what they've been eating and how frequently, because as we discussed, so many of our food decisions happen automatically.

Bringing those unconscious choices to light is so powerful. That's why I love the analysis tool I'm about to share. You can use it again and again to check in with yourself, measure your progress and get back on track when things slip (which is totally normal). What matters most is being aware of the slips and returning to your plan. I know tracking your food can be tedious, but I promise it leads to invaluable insights.

Your food diary

I'd like you to complete a food diary for at least four days, including one weekend day. You'll use the notes from your food diary to analyse and get a clearer idea of your current nutritional habits. Understanding this will help you to work through this book and track your progress.

Please fill in the diary overleaf. You should list every single food item you eat on each day.

Vegetables and fruit (V&F) Please write down the number of portions you had in that meal or snack. One portion equates to approximately one handful.

Macronutrients Please write down the number of macronutrient types you ate in that meal or snack.

— **Protein (P)** e.g. fish, meat, eggs, beans, legumes (such as lentils, chickpeas, beans), tofu, yoghurt

— **Fat (F)** e.g. cheese, butter, olive oil, avocado, coconut oil, olives, nuts, seeds

— **Carbohydrates (C)** e.g. bread, pasta, rice, quinoa, grains (such as couscous, bulgar wheat), flour, crackers, baked goods, pastries, biscuits, flapjacks

— **Processed Foods (PF)** e.g. anything that is pre-packaged and contains more than 5 ingredients on the label, with added sugar and oils

If you don't know how to categorise a food item, don't worry, just leave it out of the tally (it will become clearer as you work through the book, so you can add in later).

If a food crosses a number of categories e.g. protein and fat, log that item in the category that you believe best describes it.

Your food diary

START HERE

Day 1	Time	Food and drinks	V&F	P	F	C	PF
Breakfast							
AM snack							
Lunch							
PM snack							
Dinner							
Evening snack							
Total							

Day 2	Time	Food and drinks	V&F	P	F	C	PF
Breakfast							
AM snack							
Lunch							
PM snack							
Dinner							
Evening snack							
Total							

Day 3	Time	Food and drinks	V&F	P	F	C	PF
Breakfast							
AM snack							
Lunch							
PM snack							
Dinner							
Evening snack							
Total							

Weekend day	Time	Food and drinks	V&F	P	F	C	PF
Breakfast							
AM snack							
Lunch							
PM snack							
Dinner							
Evening snack							
Total							

Analysing your food diary

Once you've completed your food diary, you can immediately see some useful 'totals'. You'll get a quick sense of how many portions of fruit and vegetables you're currently eating each day. This is an important benchmark as we'll be working to increase your intake of these nutrient-dense foods.

The diary will also reveal your typical portions and balance of the three main macronutrients — proteins, fats and carbohydrates.

For now, don't worry about your totals, I will be explaining what the right balance is and how to achieve it. But I do want you to start the plan with these initial numbers from your food diary, as they will provide a helpful reference point as you begin to make changes.

We'll revisit these benchmarks throughout the programme to track your progress. As you go through each chapter's lessons, you can refer back to this diary and watch your totals improve. By the end, you'll be able to see clearly how your dietary patterns have transformed.

Now I'd like you to take a closer look at your food diary using a 'traffic light' system. This simple exercise will help you identify patterns and pinpoint which foods may be hindering your health. Grab three different coloured pens or highlighters (ideally, red, yellow/orange and green). Using the guide overleaf, highlight each food or drink in one of three colours:

— **Red:** to avoid/ minimise
— **Amber:** to eat in moderation
— **Green:** to eat freely

At this stage, we're using the traffic light system simply to highlight your current habits, without any judgement whatsoever.

The foods highlighted in red are ones we'll want to start phasing out over time. The amber items are foods you may need to be more mindful of portioning or pairing with fats or proteins to help balance blood sugar. The green highlighted items are foods you can feel good about eating freely.

Take a pause and simply observe the colours and patterns in your diary. Notice what areas could use some improvement, but also what you're already doing well. This analysis helps identify the next steps, while also celebrating your existing healthy habits. There's no need to change anything drastic yet. We're just bringing awareness to your current nutrition landscape.

Over the next five weeks (or more), as you work through each chapter, you'll gradually start choosing different foods and learn how to balance your plate in a way that truly nourishes your body. There's no forced deprivation or strict rules here. My aim is to empower you to choose more of the right foods and when you focus on building your plate with these foods, you will feel full and satisfied. By focusing your attention on what you should eat, over time you will naturally choose fewer of the foods you should avoid. This is an education that enables you to rediscover how to eat in a way that supports your body's needs. Your new food diary will become a visual record of that transformative journey.

Red foods

Drinks: fizzy drinks, fruit juice, shop-bought smoothies, milkshakes, diet drinks, alcoholic drinks, sports drinks, plant-based milks that contain added oils and sugars, deep-fried foods.

Ultra-processed foods: takeaway food, fast food, processed meats (bacon, ham, salami, sausage, chicken nuggets), ready meals, pre-made sauces, e.g. pasta or curry sauces, condiments (salad dressings, stir-fry sauces).

Refined carbohydrates: white bread, white pasta, white flour, white noodles, couscous, instant noodles, instant or quick porridge oats, crisps, salty snacks in a packet, breakfast cereals, cereal bars, protein bars.

Oils: sunflower oil, vegetable oil, rapeseed oil, margarines and spreads (I will be explaining why these oils are not good for you in chapter 9).

Sugar: confectionery, chocolate with less than 85 per cent cocoa solids, biscuits and cookies, flavoured yoghurts, ice cream, frozen desserts, jam, honey, marmalade, sugary spreads, artificial sweeteners.

Amber foods

Whole grains: wholegrain sourdough, wholegrain pasta, brown rice, wild rice, quinoa, bulgar wheat.

Starchy vegetables: potatoes, sweet potatoes, butternut squash, parsnips, beetroot, swede.

Dairy: milk, full-fat natural yoghurt, goat's yoghurt, cheese, butter.

Green foods

Protein: poultry, game, beef, lamb, pork, fish, eggs, beans, pulses, tofu, tempeh, full-fat Greek yoghurt.

Natural sources of fat: nuts, seeds, avocado, olives, oils, olive oil, coconut oil, avocado oil.

Non-starchy veg: asparagus, aubergine, broccoli, brussels sprouts, cabbage, cauliflower, cavolo nero, chicory, courgette, cucumber, garlic, green beans, kale, leeks, mushrooms, onions, pak choy, peppers, radish, rocket, salad leaves, spinach, swiss chard, tomatoes, watercress.

Fruit: apples, berries, kiwi, lemons and limes, melon, pears, plums (all other fruits sit in amber, see page 84 for more on why).

Spices: fresh and dried.

Herbs: fresh and dried.

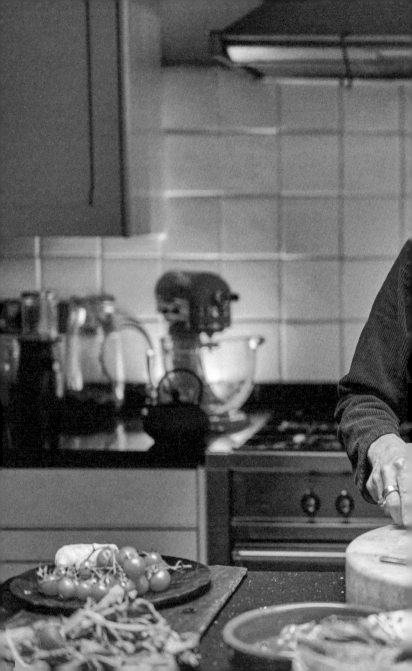

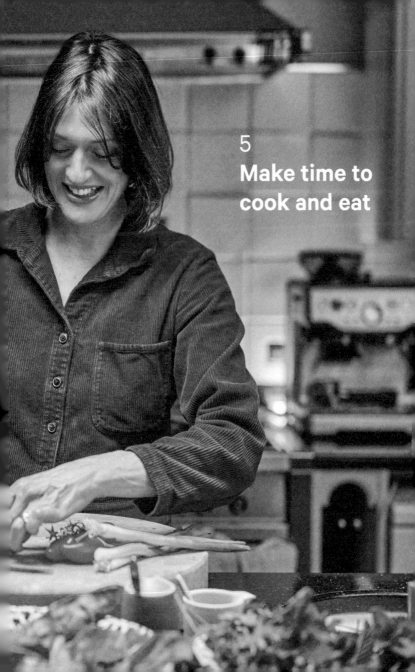

5
**Make time to
cook and eat**

What is the one thing all truly healthy people have in common? They make time to prepare and eat real food.

Preparing real food takes effort and time, yes. But it's an investment in respecting and honouring your body that allows you to live out your purpose. What is your greatest asset? It's time. And what is your most important relationship? The one you have with yourself.

Nourishment is about safeguarding your time and energy, not just today but for your future self. Taking time to cook and eat well isn't about just checking another box. It's about treating mealtimes as sacred nourishment for your mind, body and soul. How you fuel yourself impacts every aspect of your being and ability to show up fully in life. We need to be self-full, not self-ish.

The biggest barrier I hear to people changing their eating habits is, 'I don't have time to cook.' But time itself is not the issue — it's about how you prioritise your time, what's important and investing in the relationship with yourself above all else. That relationship must be non-negotiable.

When you intentionally make time for real food, you gain back exponentially more time through sustained energy, focus and disease prevention. Doing anything well requires sacrifice somewhere, you may have to give something up. The good news is that it doesn't require hours. In fact, I've found that dedicating some quality time each day to cooking can be incredibly rewarding and stress-relieving. And the commitment to it is an act of love and respect for your remarkable body. Let that be the motivation to make real food a non-negotiable priority.

Let me share some foundational practices that I have seen really work to build a consistent, enjoyable cooking habit. I use these strategies in clinic and in my own kitchen.

Cooking hour
First things first, schedule a daily 'cooking hour' and treat it like a non-negotiable appointment with yourself. Block off 30–60 minutes in your calendar and make this your cooking window. When that time shows up, drop everything else and get ready to cook. Trust me, the world won't end if you hit pause on emails or chores for a little while.

Cook once to eat twice
Get in the habit of cooking once to eat twice. Whenever you're preparing a meal, double the recipe so you've got leftovers ready for lunch the next day. It's a huge timesaver and ensures you always have options.

Enjoy this time
Make your cooking hour enjoyable! Play your favourite music, set the tone with some candles or mood lighting to create a space you want to spend time in. You've carved out this time to unwind from life's busyness and reconnect with yourself, so make sure you do.

Be flexible

Now, I get it, life can be unpredictable. Some days, your cooking hour might get disrupted by unexpected curveballs. That's okay. Embrace the flexibility and know that you can always adjust. The important thing is making the conscious effort to prioritise this time for yourself. So, I encourage you to start exploring what a dedicated daily cooking hour could look like for you. Be flexible and forgiving as you integrate this new ritual. But most importantly, show up for yourself consistently.

If you already dedicate time to preparing nourishing meals — well done. Keep doing what you are doing.

Savour the pace

> To eat is human, to digest is divine.
> Mark Twain

Food is one of life's greatest pleasures, am I right? The experience of savouring a delicious meal is hard-wired into our very being. Way back when our survival depended on seeking out nourishing foods, our brilliant brains evolved to flood us with feel-good neurotransmitters like dopamine whenever we consumed something tasty. But let's be honest, when was the last time you really allowed yourself to fully feel and experience that pleasure?

I'm talking about truly tasting and experiencing every single bite instead of mindlessly placing food into your mouth while distracted by work, the TV or rushing out the door. So many of us just aren't present enough to experience the satisfaction that nourishing ourselves can provide.

By simply slowing down and savouring each mouthful, you engage all your senses better. You'll start to notice the flavours, textures and aromas in more detail as you eat mindfully. It allows you to fully enjoy the pure pleasure of the experience.

But there's more. When you eat slowly and stay present during mealtimes, chewing properly, it aids your digestion by thoroughly breaking the food down into the smallest particles and increasing the surface area on which digestive enzymes can act, while also enhancing nutrient absorption. Chewing properly enables your digestion to work at full capacity and transport nutrients where they're needed, to regulate blood sugar adeptly and keep you feeling energised.

Through my work with many clients struggling with digestive issues, I've seen just how profound the impact of simply adjusting the pace at which they eat can be. What may seem like a minor tweak ends up resulting in massive improvements to their gut health and overall wellbeing.

As we get older, our digestive system often doesn't work quite as efficiently as it did in our younger years. A variety of factors can come into play, leading to a decline in the production of the crucial stomach juices and digestive enzymes that help us break down foods properly. When that happens, we become more susceptible to issues like poor nutrient absorption, bacterial overgrowth in the gut and uncomfortable inflammation. But with a little extra care and intention around how and what we're eating; we can help support our digestion.

Eating slowly also allows you to tune into your body's natural signals of satiety or feeling full. You'll recognise far better when you've had just enough instead of mindlessly overeating past the point of fullness.

Something I love to do with clients is to practise this with chocolate. Grab a piece of dark chocolate with around 75–85 per cent cacao. Find a comfortable, distraction-free spot in your home to settle into for about 5 minutes. This is also a great tool if you are feeling a little stressed or frazzled.

Begin by taking a few grounding breaths to relax your body and mind, preparing yourself to fully experience the taste. Set a timer for 5 minutes, then pick up the chocolate. Rather than immediately indulging, pause to appreciate its appearance — look at the rich colours, its sheen and texture. Breathe in the aroma through your nostrils, allowing any mouth-watering sensations to arise.

When you're ready, gently place the chocolate on your tongue. Instead of biting into it, keep your mouth closed and resist that instinctive urge to chew. Let the chocolate slowly melt, coating your tongue. Close your eyes if you like, tuning into the flavours and textures as it dissolves. Notice the bitterness, sweetness and velvety mouthfeel as it transitions from solid to warm liquid. See if you can detect hints of fruitiness, nuttiness, or that distinctive cacao flavour.

When the chocolate has fully melted away reflect on your experience. Wasn't that single square of chocolate more pleasurable?

So, think of 'going slower' during mealtimes not as wasted time, but as a powerful investment in your own health and fulfilment. When you fuel yourself with that level of unhurried presence, you're giving your body the gift of pleasure and optimal functioning.

Here are my tips for eating slower:

— **Allow at least 15–20 minutes to eat your meals,** or longer if possible.

— **Sit at a table away from all distractions** like TV, phones or computers.

— **Make mealtimes a sacred ritual.** Remember that nourishing yourself is an act of self-care. Each meal presents an opportunity to experience pleasure while making you stronger.

— **Before taking that first bite, pause to appreciate your plate of food.** Notice the colours, contemplate where the ingredients came from and how they reached your table. Allow your senses to awaken as saliva begins pooling in your mouth.

— **When you do start eating, take one modest mouthful at a time.** Engage mindfully by chewing each bite slowly at least 10 times, or aim for 30 chews to fully experience the flavours and textures.

— **Between bites, place your utensils down completely.** This helps reset your attention and prevents hurried shovelling of food.

You understand the science, you're making time to cook and eat slowly. Get ready to start your 6-week plan to nourish your body and mind.

Part two — Your 6-week plan to nourish

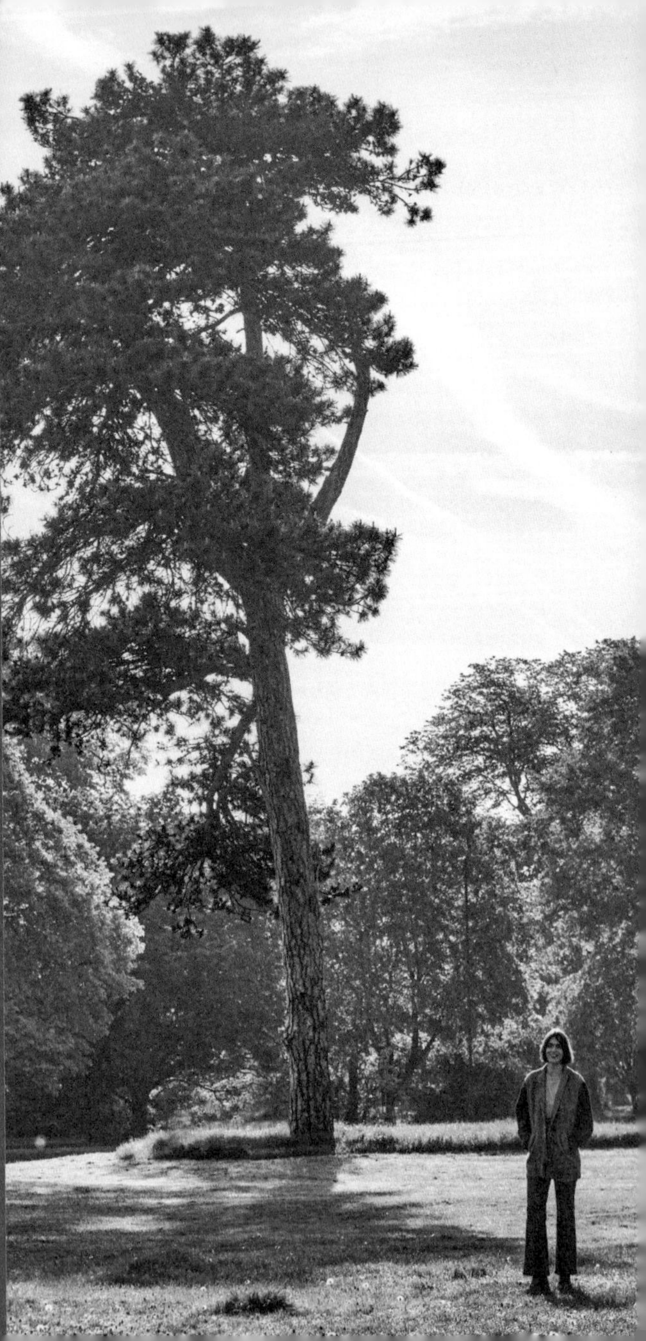

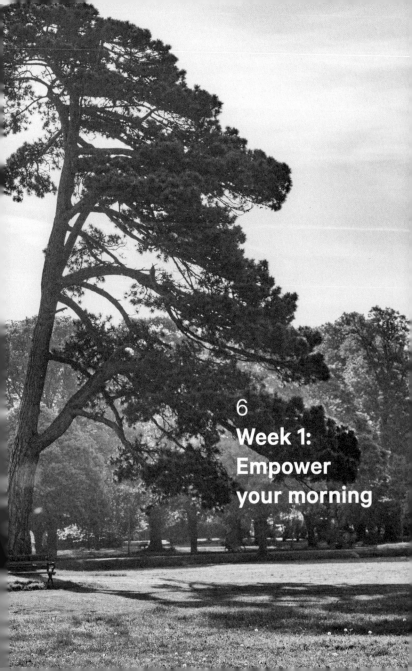

6
**Week 1:
Empower
your morning**

> In the end, it's not the years in your life that count, it's the life in your years.

Oliver Burkeman, *Four Thousand Weeks*

These days, we're constantly seeking ways to boost our energy levels. However, the energy equation is not as simple as: energy in = energy out. Despite consuming sufficient calories, many of us still struggle with persistent fatigue and a lack of vitality.

The quest for energy efficiency is about achieving a delicate balance between external demands and our energy supply. While proper nutrition plays a role, energy is about more than just nutritional intake. Stress, lack of sleep and excessive worries all affect our energy levels and can force your body's energy system into overdrive, with extra stress hormones burning through your energy reserves too quickly and disrupting your body's natural rhythms. Consequently, you may feel persistently depleted and your body's ability to regulate blood sugar levels can become compromised.

Energy is also a feeling, a state of being that you have control over. It's something you can actively create for yourself: you generate positive energy through self-efficacy and personal empowerment. This begins with cultivating the right mindset from the start of the day — by waking up well and how you approach each morning.

Change the way you wake up

Think back to this morning. What's the first thing you did when you woke up? Did you pick up your phone, check social media or your emails? It's easy to do. But almost immediately, your day would have begun to fill up with tasks and a to-do list, maybe even stress (depending on who the email was from!). Your brain would already have been thinking about what was ahead, yet you hadn't even stepped out of bed. Your mind, mood and motivation had been hijacked.

But you can choose a different way to start the day. By intentionally guiding your mornings and prioritising self-care, you can preserve and even boost your energy. Instead of immediately depleting your mental resources on emails and tasks, you can channel that energy into activities that set a positive tone for the day.

I'm not suggesting you spend lots of time reading in bed, but you could make a small change or a new daily habit. It doesn't have to be complex: go for a short walk, write a page in a journal, read a chapter of a book, do some breathwork, meditate for 10 minutes or simply get straight into the shower or bath and focus on some self-care as you take that time for yourself. Do something that makes you feel good, resist the urge to go online for at least the first hour of your morning; better yet for 2 hours. By doing so, you are not just avoiding early morning stress, you are actively building up mental and physical reserves. This intentional start allows you to approach your tasks with more focus and resilience, making you more efficient and effective throughout the day. Waking up well is more than just feeling good; it's an act of self-empowerment that enriches your life and enhances your overall productivity.

Get natural daylight in the morning

Our bodies operate according to a circadian clock, a complex internal system that regulates our natural sleep/wake cycle. This biological timekeeper plays a crucial role in determining our energy, motivation and focus for the day (plus much more).

The circadian clock is primarily regulated by light and dark cycles, but it's also significantly influenced by nutrition and stress. When functioning optimally, the system ensures that you wake up feeling refreshed, energetic and mentally alert, so by aligning your morning routine with your body's natural rhythms, you will be setting yourself up for optimal performance and wellbeing throughout the day.

In the morning your body needs to build up specific hormones and neurotransmitters involved in wakefulness; one critical hormone involved in this process is cortisol. Cortisol is often associated with bad stress, but in fact we need it at the right time of the day. When you see daylight outside, your circadian clock sends out signals (peptides, hormones, but also neural signals) to the brain and body saying, 'Hey, now it's daytime, be fully awake.' Cortisol peaks usually about 30 minutes after waking. These signals also trigger the release of serotonin (your happy neurotransmitter) and dopamine (your motivator hormone), which have a direct line to the structures of the brain associated with mood and motivation. Getting outside first thing and seeing natural daylight (safely with no sunglasses) is a simple yet powerful way to support this process. This habit can help improve your energy, mood and focus.

Neuroscientist Andrew Huberman has revealed that exposure to bright morning sunlight results in a 50 per cent increase in the natural morning cortisol spike, which is a good thing.

Try to get at least 30 minutes of midday sun too. The more natural sunlight you get outside during the day the better, assuming you are doing this safely. Accessing natural daylight in the middle of the day is also important to help stimulate melatonin synthesis (our sleep hormone).

Fuel your morning

When it comes to nutrition, three key areas lay the foundation for a well-set day:

1. Drink more water in the daytime

Your brain is on average made up of 80 per cent water, which is even more prevalent than your body, which is made up of about 60 per cent water. Water is nutrition; your body cannot store water, you need a fresh supply every day to make up the losses that occur from functioning.

Dehydration occurs when you use lose more water than you take in. Your body is constantly using and losing water, especially during sleep, when your brain and body tap into your water supply to restore, rejuvenate and detoxify. Even as little as a 1–2 per cent decrease in water intake immediately affects the brain's fluid balance, leading to fatigue, mood swings, headaches and making it difficult to focus and make decisions. In the UK, the average adult drinks approximately half of what their body needs.

Researchers in the UK conducted an experiment to test the potential effects of water on cognitive performance and mood. They had the participants complete a series of mental tests after eating a cereal bar. Some participants consumed the cereal bar alone; the rest were also given water to drink. Those who drank three cups of water just before completing the test showed significantly faster reaction times compared to those who didn't.

Think about the benefits of thinking faster, improving memory, coordination, focus and mood. Before you reach for your morning coffee, prioritise hydration. Start your day by drinking a large glass (240ml) of water before you do anything, and if you can manage two glasses, even better. Notice how you feel when you are truly hydrated; pay attention to how your brain feels, your energy and mood.

Throughout the day aim to drink approximately one glass of water each hour. The body's circadian clock regulates the cells within the kidneys so, during the daytime, the kidneys work efficiently to filter fluid, then output reduces while you are asleep, so that hopefully you do not frequently wake up during the night to urinate!

2. Delay your morning caffeine boost

Do you struggle with that afternoon slump?

Waiting a bit for that first cup of coffee can make a big difference to your energy in the afternoon. Caffeine makes you feel awake by intercepting adenosine — a molecule that signals sleepiness. As the day progresses, adenosine builds up, nudging you towards sleep in the evening, and helping you get a good night's sleep. It clears out once you sleep. Caffeine blocks adenosine receptors, preventing the sleepy build-up.

When you wake up in the morning your adenosine levels are at their lowest. Delaying that caffeine kick by around 90 minutes lets your body wake up naturally, aiding your natural cortisol flow.

Drinking your caffeine when you are fully awake and alert allows your body to wake up naturally without disrupting your natural sleep/wake cycle. You will also enjoy it more as you may be craving it a little.

Caffeine has approximately a 5-hour half-life, i.e. half of the dose will still be in your system five hours later. By delaying your caffeine intake, you are working with your body's natural rhythm, amplifying that natural morning cortisol peak and delaying the adenosine build-up in the afternoon that may be driving the slump. Enjoy one cup of coffee in the morning 90 minutes after waking. Do not drink any caffeine after midday as not to interrupt sleep.

Too much caffeine can be a bad thing as caffeine is also a mild stressor and can be addictive. If you struggle with sleep, I recommend removing caffeine altogether as it is associated with disrupted sleep — either difficulty falling asleep or waking in the night.

3. Breaking your fast

Breakfast is more than just a meal; it's about breaking your overnight fast, therefore your first meal of the day is the most vital to effectively fuel your body with the essential nutrients for optimal functioning. Whether you identify as a breakfast eater or not, the first meal in your day theoretically breaks your overnight fast.

There's an old saying that holds true: 'Eat breakfast like a king, lunch like a prince, and dinner like a pauper.' Research supports the positive impact of having a substantial morning meal to support healthy sleep/wake cycles, fat burning and overall health. While making breakfast the largest meal in the day may not always be feasible, focusing on its quality is possible and vital.

Avoid starting your day with a blood sugar spike that will inevitably be followed by an energy-draining crash that disrupts your mood, appetite and focus.

Balancing your blood sugar by eating the right foods can positively influence how you feel immediately after breakfast, as well as stabilising your energy levels throughout the day.

In reality, the first meal of the day can pose challenges. Convenient, widespread choices like shop-bought cereals and granola, protein bars, instant porridge, muesli or seemingly healthy smoothies can resemble desserts more than a nutritious breakfast. Many of these are highly processed foods that contain sugars, additives, emulsifiers and sweeteners that can adversely affect mood, energy and immunity. These foods deliver empty calories and are high in carbohydrates that wreck your metabolism for the rest of the day.

Let's transform your breakfast routine with these essentials:

Make breakfast count
Kick-start your day with a nourishing breakfast. This can be at the time you feel hungry, which might mean waiting a bit. However, studies have shown that eating earlier in the day may be better for how your body handles food, for your overall metabolic health and for keeping your energy levels balanced across the day.

Choose real food
Say no to ultra-processed breakfast options (check labels), such as cereals, cereal bars, shop-bought granola, protein bars, sweetened yoghurt, shop-bought juice, shop-bought smoothies, instant porridge, processed bread, bagels, pastries and pancakes (refer back to your traffic light table and pick from the options opposite for healthy alternatives).

Make your breakfast at home

It's best to prepare your breakfast at home and avoid buying a takeaway breakfast, so if you are working and would rather eat breakfast later, consider bringing it to work for a healthier start to your day.

Prioritise protein

Ensure your breakfast includes a good source of protein. At first simply aim to include some protein in your breakfast, then as you get used to this you can begin to look at increasing the amount. Starting your day with protein will help you to reach your protein requirement for the day as many people struggle to do this. Protein is also the most satiating macronutrient and helps to balance blood sugar to keep energy stable. Your neurotransmitters are built from proteins, so feed your brain (there's lots more about protein in the next chapter and breakfast recipes on page 143).

Try these healthy options:

— **Full-fat Greek yoghurt with 2 tablespoons of chia seeds or hemp seeds, berries and topped with a few nuts** (option to stir in a good-quality protein powder or collagen powder to increase the protein)

— **Swiss chard or spinach with soft-boiled or poached eggs with full-fat Greek yoghurt**

— **3 soft-boiled or poached eggs, smoked salmon, tomatoes and spinach**

— **Omelette (made with 3 soft-boiled or poached eggs) with spinach and rocket salad**

— **Sardines with spinach and tomatoes**

- **Chia seed overnight oats with blueberries** (see recipe page 144)

- **Grain-free porridge** (see recipe page 143)

- **Homemade granola** (see recipe page 147) and full-fat Greek yoghurt

- **Green protein smoothie** (see page 141 for my guide to making this)

As well as breaking your fast with a healthy breakfast option, it's equally important to consider when you eat your last meal of the day and how this affects your body. We all practise fasting when we sleep at night. Digestion is energy-intensive and having a full gut can hinder the body's ability to heal and rest. When you have no food in your digestive tract it allows your body to focus on repair. In an ideal world your last meal would be 2–3 hours before you go to bed.

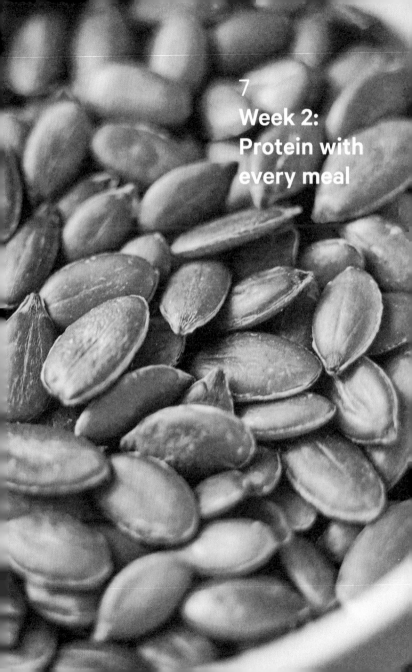

7
**Week 2:
Protein with
every meal**

Protein is the foundation of life. Every cell in your body depends on it for structure, function and repair. It's not just about muscular; it's about the intricate machinery that keeps you alive and thriving.

Dr Bruce Ames

Your breakfast is taken care of and you're waking up with energy. For week two, let's focus on protein.

One of the things some of my clients get a bit nervous about when making changes to their food is feeling hungry. That's why we are going to focus on protein first. Protein is incredibly satiating and the most important macronutrient. When clients increase their protein, they are always surprised by how much longer they can go without feeling hungry between meals, and it helps to reduce cravings.

While protein is brilliant for promoting fullness, it offers benefits that go far beyond just fighting off hunger. Protein is a multi-talented essential macronutrient crucial for optimising your body's overall function and wellbeing. It helps sustain steady energy levels throughout the day, keeps your metabolism efficient and is absolutely vital in preserving muscle mass and bone strength.

Protein acts as a building block. It is made up of chains called amino acids. There are 20 different amino acids in total, 9 of which are considered 'essential' because your body cannot produce them on its own; you must obtain them from the foods you eat. These chains construct components throughout your body, from creating brand new cells to repairing ageing ones. Protein provides that strong structural scaffolding for bones, ligaments, tendons and even makes up parts of major organs like your liver, brain and skin.

But protein's role extends even further. It controls various critical bodily functions by forming enzymes that speed up and regulate countless chemical reactions in your body. It is also essential for constructing the neurotransmitters that regulate mood, cognition, motivation and focus and plays a pivotal role in balancing hormones and in building and maintaining your immune system.

As you get older, your levels of gastric juices can decline, making it harder for your body to absorb protein from food, a condition called 'maldigestion', and your body becomes less efficient at building and maintaining muscle. At around age 40, you start losing a significant portion of lean muscle mass — about 8 per cent per decade, according to Dr Donald Layman, a researcher in the field of nutrition known for his work on protein, metabolism and health. This puts you at a greater risk of sarcopenia (muscle wasting), brittle bones and fractures.

Maintaining good muscle health is key for optimal resilience. Having adequate muscle mass is essential to stabilise blood sugar and enable the body to utilise energy efficiently. The more muscle mass you have, the better your insulin sensitivity, as muscle tissue serves as a significant reservoir for glucose. Remember that insulin's role is to send glucose into cells (acting like a key to unlock the door of the cells). With more muscle mass, muscle cells can absorb more glucose, reducing the amount stored in the liver or fat cells. Therefore, muscle mass is integral for optimal blood sugar management and overall health resilience.

Here's a quick summary of all the benefits of eating protein:

— **Balances blood sugar**

— **Reduces cravings, keeps you feeling fuller for longer**

— **Has been shown to improve body composition**

— **Helps maintain and increase muscle mass**
(muscles are your biggest glucose sink)

— **Supports mental clarity**

— **Increases energy**

— **Keeps bones strong**

— **Reduces the risk of sarcopenia and osteoporosis**

To maintain proper intake, the recommended daily amount is 0.8 grams of protein per kilogram of body weight. This doesn't account for activity level or specific metabolic needs like recovering from an illness. As mentioned, as you age and become less efficient at processing protein, individuals over 40 should aim to consume 1.4–1.8 grams per kilogram of body weight. If you are physically active, it is best to aim for the higher end of that range.

Most of the research shows that getting 20–30 grams of ingested protein per meal is the ideal to maximise muscle protein synthesis — the process through which your body builds and maintains lean muscle mass by using protein. I favour the higher end of this to promote satiety and manage blood sugar.

The key is to space out your protein intake throughout the day into 3–4 meals or snacks, rather than trying to cram it all into just one or two sittings. That way, your body has a steady supply of amino acids to pull from.

For now, your goal should be to make sure you have a solid portion of protein at breakfast, lunch and dinner. Don't stress about weighing or calculating grams. A good rule of thumb is to aim for 1–2 palm-sized portions of a protein-rich food. If you're eating protein consistently with your meals, you're on the right track. You can fine-tune the quantities based on the above calculation once you're eating it consistenly. But first, just get into the habit of making protein a part of your breakfast, lunch and dinner routine. You've started with breakfast, so now we'll work on balancing your other meals.

When it comes to getting all those essential amino acids your body needs, animal-based proteins are called 'complete' sources. That means they contain all 9 of the essential amino acids in sufficient quantities to meet your needs in just one serving. Eggs, poultry and fish are the best sources of amino acids.

Some plant proteins, on the other hand, are considered 'incomplete' proteins. While they do contain some of the essential amino acids, typically they are low or missing one or more of them. If you follow a vegan nutrition plan, you'll want to be mindful of combining different plant protein sources to ensure you get that complete amino acid profile. My recommendation for vegan clients is to choose complete plant proteins where you can (see the table on page 75 for examples) and to pair legumes like beans or lentils with some nuts or seeds. That complementary combo provides all the essential aminos your body needs to thrive.

When choosing animal protein sources, prioritise unprocessed or minimally processed options. Avoid highly processed meats like bacon, sausages and salami and opt for grass-fed. For soy-based proteins, traditional Asian varieties like edamame, miso, tofu and tempeh are preferable to many Western soy products, such as soy-based burgers, soy-based meat alternatives and cheeses which may be genetically modified and contain additives. Opt for organic, fermented soy foods where possible.

By choosing organic you can avoid the potential health and environmental risks associated with GMOs (genetically modified organisms) and pesticides, which are commonly prevalent in soy production.

Your protein cheat sheet

The table shows you how much of a food item you need to consume to get approximately 30g of protein. All weights listed are the cooked weight.

There are some foods opposite that can help you meet your protein goal more easily, for example, animal proteins and organic soy proteins. Others foods listed can be used to help you top up your protein amounts, for example adding an egg to a meal, eating a serving of Greek yoghurt with nuts and seeds as dessert, or topping salads or veggies with nuts and seeds.

---

1 organic grass-fed whey protein with no added sugars, colourings, flavourings, artificial flavours or gums (no ingredient names you aren't familiar with, see appendix on page 144)

2 with no added sugars, colourings, flavourings, artificial flavours or gums (no ingredient names you aren't familiar with, see appendix on page 144)

Produce	Approx. serving size
Animal protein (ideally organic, grass-fed, wild)	
Sardines	120g
Salmon	112g
White fish	125g
Chicken	120g
Turkey mince	120g
Lean steak	107g
Lean mince	136g
Lamb chop	110g
Eggs	4
Whey protein powders[1]	1–2 scoops
Plant protein	
Tempeh (organic) (complete protein —contains all essential amino acids)	150g
Tofu (organic) (complete protein)	170g
Lentils	340g
Beans/legumes (tinned)	340g
Edamame beans	250g
Quinoa (complete protein)	375g
Plant protein powder[2]	1–2 scoops

Dairy and organic soy yoghurt are great ways to top up your protein.

Here is what one portion approximately provides in protein:

Portion	Protein
150g Greek yoghurt	10g of protein
150g organic soy yoghurt	7g of protein
150g cottage cheese[3]	17g of protein

Here are the protein amounts per 1 tablespoon serving for seeds and nuts. Nuts and seeds are another great way to top up your protein intake each meal.

1 tablespoon serving	Protein
Chia seeds (complete protein)	2g
Hemp seed hearts (complete protein)	3g
Pumpkin seeds	2g
Sunflower seeds	2g
Peanuts	4g
Almonds	3g

---

3   this is the type of cheese with the most protein; other cheeses are considered to be a fat source (see chapter 9)

Let's look at your protein using a simple framework.

First, take a look at your typical daily meals. Are you including a protein source with each of them — breakfast, lunch and dinner? If not, that's an easy win.

Reference the list of protein options and find one or two you can start incorporating into the meals that are currently lacking protein.

Next, look at your portion sizes. Ideally, you want to aim for 1–2 palm-sized servings of your protein source per meal (this is a way to review how much you are eating without weighing your food), so visually size that up. If your protein option looks small (smaller than the size of your palm), there's room for increasing it a bit to hit that target. If you are struggling with cravings, eating a vegan diet, looking to improve body composition or muscle mass, or are training, aim for two palm-sized portions.

And if even after increasing your main protein, you're still falling short, look for ways to add a little boost. Throw some seeds or nuts on a salad or have some Greek yoghurt at the end of your meal.

Don't overcomplicate it; it's just about protein awareness with each eating opportunity, and making simple adjustments to your current eating habits by choosing the protein sources you enjoy. At this stage there is no need to weigh your food. Here are some quick protein tips to help:

When planning out your meals and snacks, make protein the priority. Think about what your protein source will be.

Get organised by making a list of protein-rich foods you enjoy eating. Having your favourites written down helps with meal planning.

Stock up those protein staples when shopping.
Having a variety of fresh, frozen and tinned options
at home makes it easier to include protein.

Don't forget to eat protein at breakfast.

If a meal plan is looking a little protein light,
look for simple ways to boost it:

— Use a full-fat natural Greek yoghurt to make salad
dressing; add some to soups, or curries, or enjoy
with berries.

— Mix cottage cheese, tofu or organic soy yoghurt into
dishes like curries, soups and stews, or serve as a side.

— Add beans, lentils or chicken to salads.

— Sauté tempeh or tofu and toss into stir-fries, salads
or soups.

— Swap rice for quinoa or lentils.

— Use silken tofu (a soft, delicate type of tofu with a
smooth custard-like texture) to make creamy sauces
for curries and stews.

— Make a vegetable frittata or omelette to have as a
quick option.

— Top soups, stews, salads with 2 cooked eggs.

— Add in a protein smoothie as a snack or serve
alongside a meal.

— Sprinkle nuts and seeds on salads or veggie sides.

You can also consider batch cooking and prepping several protein sources all at once.

— Pick your proteins and season them with spices and rubs (see page 121).

— Cook them all at the same time using your preferred method. Portion into individual servings then refrigerate or put in the freezer.

— Cook meals like stews and curries in large quantities; prepare hard-boiled eggs in batches to store in the fridge, or make a frittata.

— Roasted fish also keeps well for a quick salad the next day.

— Alternatively, simple double your dinner quantity when you cook so that you have something for lunch the next day.

If you're someone who travels a lot, invest in some quality food storage containers and an insulated lunch bag — that way your proteins and meals are easy to transport.

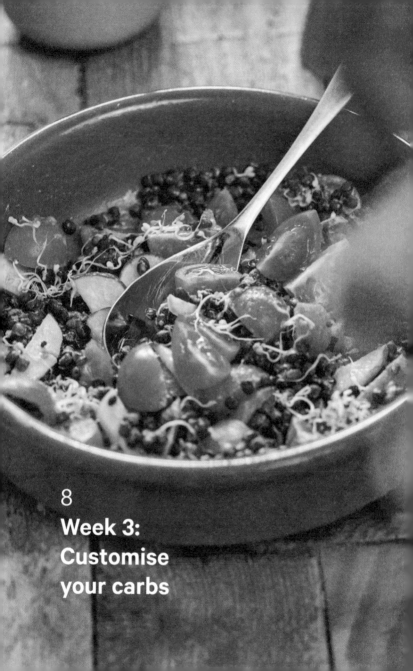

8
**Week 3:
Customise
your carbs**

Carbohydrates are made up of glucose molecules, the nutrients found in foods that provide sugar, starch and fibre. You're likely well aware that not all carbohydrates are created equal — the type of carbohydrate you consume can have vastly different effects on your body. This is because they come in two main forms: simple and complex.

Simple carbs are those found in sweets, refined grains (such as white bread and white pasta), juices and smoothies. They are digested quickly and can cause a rapid spike in blood sugar levels. If your body can efficiently regulate these fluctuations, the spike may not pose a problem, however, for many it can be problematic leading to the complications mentioned in chapter 3 (see pages 32–33).

Then you've got complex carbs, the ones packed with fibre (such as brown rice, brown pasta, oats; starchy vegetables like sweet potatoes and butternut squash; and legumes, such as beans and lentils). These take a bit more effort to break down, leading to a slower, more gradual rise in blood sugar, allowing your cells to absorb the sugar steadily, in a controlled way, without the peaks and crashes. This leaves less excess to be stored as fat or build up in your liver. We'll look at fibre in more detail in chapter 10.

Your body can make all the glucose it needs through a process called gluconeogenesis; therefore, carbs are considered as non-essential. While your body can make glucose, some glucose from the right sources can be benefical for brain function and physical activity.

Most UK adults are getting between 46–52 per cent of their calories from carbohydrates. I've shared this not to emphasise the calorie aspect, but because it suggests a potential overconsumption of this one nutrient source at the expense of undereating essential nutrients your cells need. The science points to a reasonable intake of approximately 80–100 grams of carbohydrate a day. However, the typical UK adult is eating approximately 250–300 grams of carbohydrate per day. Our bodies are not designed to eat that quantity in a single day and overconsumption of simple carbs can lead to issues like carbohydrate intolerance and blood sugar dysregulation.

You can absolutely enjoy carbs by choosing high-fibre complex carbs and being mindful of the amount you eat in one meal. Other foods matter much more (you've just learned about protein and will learn more as you progress through this book). High-fibre complex carbs can help satisfy your hunger and make you feel full, while simple carb sources may actually increase hunger and cravings. Studies show that eating a high-carb breakfast leads to hunger returning sooner compared to a lower-carb and higher-fat/protein breakfast. Protein takes longer to digest and helps you feel fuller and more satisfied for a longer period of time; I will share more about fats in the next chapter.

The quantity of carbs you can consume to keep your blood glucose in a healthy range is unique to you —

everyone's tolerance level is different, which adds a layer of complexity. You may be able to manage and metabolise carbs effectively, avoiding adverse blood sugar spikes, or you may need to keep your intake lower. Your age, health status, physical activity levels, gender and if you are taking medications will all play some part in how well you metabolise carbs. This is referred to as your carbohydrate tolerance.

One of the best ways to determine your carbohydrate tolerance and what is going on with your insulin and blood glucose is to wear a continuous glucose monitor (CGM) for a week or two. It's a great way to track you blood sugar response in real time, to understand better how carbs affect you. However, you don't need to have a CGM to find your carbohydrate tolerance. You can play detective and feel the impact of a blood sugar spike by paying attention to how you feel after you eat. If you feel tired, agitated, crave sugar or caffeine, find it difficult to focus, or even experience anxiety, that is a message from your body that you have eaten something that is not good for you. You can then begin to investigate and adjust your food.

Your goal this week is to look at the quality and the quantity of carbohydrates that you are eating in meals to find your carbohydrate tolerance.

Let's start with quality

Begin by removing refined carbohydrate sources, as these foods cause the biggest glucose spikes (they are in red on your traffic light system, see page 48) and swap to healthier versions. You'll find suggestions on page 86.

Be aware of foods that are high in starch or may contain hidden sugars which increase blood sugar levels. These include:

— Most plant milk substitutes — look at the label as many have added sugar and oils
— Dried fruit snacks, marketed as healthy
— Protein bars and protein powders
— Pasta sauces, curry sauces and most pre-made shop-bought sauces
— Popcorn, puffed rice, other puffed grains
— Processed gluten-free baked products
— Soups
— Alcohol

Hidden sugars

Hidden sugars can be found in various forms on food labels. Here are some common names to look out for and avoid:

— sucrose
— fructose
— glucose
— starchy hydrolysates
— maltose
— dextrose
— corn syrup

— high fructose corn syrup
— fruit juice concentrate
— caramel
— maltodextrin
— sorghum syrup
— barley syrup
— rice syrup

What about fruit?

Fruits are considered a carbohydrate-rich food and they contain natural sugars. It's important to know that not all fruit contains the same amount of sugar. Some are higher in natural sugars. Choose 1 or 2 portions of fruit per day and opt for the lower sugar options; these are listed as green in the traffic light system. I would also recommend combining the low sugar fruit with a healthy fat, for example a handful of nuts or some full-fat Greek yoghurt, to slow the rate at which the sugars are absorbed into the bloodstream.

What carbs to choose

If you choose to eat carbs, swap to unrefined carbohydrates that are minimally processed, i.e. as close as possible to their natural state. These foods include:

— **Brown rice**
— **Wild rice**
— **Quinoa**
— **Soba noodles**
— **Beans, pulses and lentils**
— **Sweet potatoes** (starchy veg)
— **Butternut squash** (starchy veg)
— **Jumbo or steel-cut oats**
— **Seed crackers**
— **Pasta alternatives** (see table on page 86)
— **If you are using flour** in your cooking opt for wholegrain versions or substitute with coconut flour or almond flour
— **If you choose to eat bread** opt for a brown sourdough
— **Seed-based breads**

How to swap bad to good carbs

You can find great alternatives to foods that you may love and be worried about removing. There are so many great alternatives now to help you make better choices for the longer term. Below is a guide to some swaps.

Replace	Healthy alternatives
Bread and crackers	Seed breads and seeded crackers Some good brands include: — Keto 8, *8foods.co.uk* — Dillon Organic, *dillonorganic.co.uk* — Sunshine Organic Bakery
Granola	Homemade (see recipe on page 147)
Pasta	Lentil pasta, edamame pasta, chickpea pasta
White rice	Quinoa Beans and lentils Brown or wild rice Broccoli rice or cauliflower rice
Crisps	Nuts and seeds
Sweets	Dark chocolate (85 per cent cocoa solids — work your way up to this) Low-sugar fruits — apples, berries, melon, citrus fruits and plums
Noodles made from white flour	Soba noodles Buckwheat noodles
White flour	Wholegrain versions or substitute with coconut flour or almond flour

Find your balance

Quantity is very individual as mentioned. It's recognised that limiting your carbohydrate intake to around 30 grams per meal, equivalent to approximately one cupped handful, effectively helps to prevent blood sugar spikes and insulin surges when your carbs are eaten with non-starchy vegetables, protein and healthy fats. A golden rule is never to eat carbs alone. If you are balancing your plate well (with protein, veggies and healthy fats) you may not need that much carbohydrate.

Personalising your carbohydrate intake requires a bit of experimentation to find your balance. Now that you know which carbs to choose, I suggest that you start by eating the recommended one cupped handful per meal. Monitor how you feel after meals in a food diary. Use this as a baseline, and gradually experiment with increasing or reducing your carbohydrate intake. Your body can produce all the glucose it needs, so don't worry about consuming enough. Your body can also utilise fat for energy too, and will do this when carbs are lower.

Take one step at a time, beginning with one meal. Small steps help you build a solid understanding of your body's responses.

1. **Choose quality carbs:**
— Know the difference between refined and unrefined (go back to the list on page 85).
— Swap your current choices for better options.

2. **Review your frequency of carb consumption:**
— Assess how often you include carbs in your day.
— Avoid snacking on carbs.
— Never eat carbs alone.

3. Assess your carb quantity and find your tolerance level:
— Reduce intake to one cupped handful per meal.
— Diarise how you feel after you eat.
— Adjust levels accordingly.

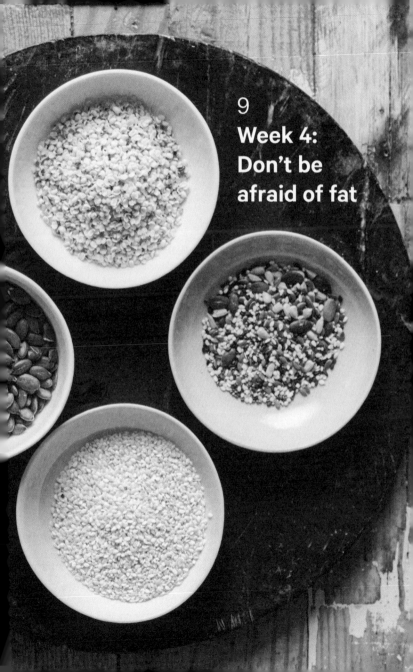

9

Week 4:
Don't be
afraid of fat

A fat is not a fat.

Dr Robert Lustig

Dietary fat, or the fat we eat from food, is probably one of the most controversial areas of nutrition. It's a tale of shifting science, marketing opinions and fearmongering, all of which drive cultural anxiety. It's complex but I am going to try and keep it simple, so buckle up.

The fear surrounding dietary fat largerly stems from its association with cholesterol and heart disease. For decades the prevailing belief was that eating dietary fat, especially saturated fat, directly increased blood cholesterol levels, leading to an increased risk of heart disease. This oversimplified view led to widespread fat-phobia and the promotion of low-fat diets.

However, recent research has shown that the relationship between dietary fat, cholesterol and heart disease is much more nuanced. While cholesterol is found in some fatty foods, dietary cholesterol dosen't necessarily translate directly to blood cholesterol levels for most people.

Cholesterol is a type of fat that is often misunderstood. We all need cholesterol to survive — it's a special kind of fat that your body needs to stay healthy and you'll find it in every cell in your body. Cholesterol is crucial for many bodily functions: it helps build your cell walls, makes hormones and keeps your brain working properly. In fact, your brain has more cholesterol than any other part of your body and it's vital for your neurotransmitters. It's that important that your body can make it.

Understanding cholesterol is especially important if you're in your 40s or if heart disease or diabetes runs in your family. Heart disease often develops silently, so grasping the basics can help you navigate your health, understand your risk factors, and actively build resilience. I believe everyone should have a better understanding of this information and at the very least know their key metabolic health markers to be able to better understand their risk (see Testing on pages 136–140).

The two areas I suspect you worry about the most are: will eating fat make you fat? Will consuming saturated fat or cholesterol increase your risk of heart disease? I am hoping to give you peace of mind by debunking some myths and looking at the current scientific thinking.

Cholesterol: a more complex tale than we thought

You've likely heard the terms 'good cholesterol' (HDL-C) and 'bad cholesterol' (LDL-C). It turns out not all LDL cholesterol is the same — there are large and small particles. The small, dense LDL-C particles are more troublesome than the large ones as they can get into your artery walls and cause problems, including heart disease.

The delicate lining of your blood vessels is called the endothelium and can be damaged by various factors:

— Smoking
— High blood pressure (often linked to high blood sugar)
— High blood sugar

When these vessels are unhealthy, small dense LDL-C particles are more likely to get trapped in them. But it seems that sugar and refined carbs might be the real culprit behind heart disease, potentially increasing the small LDL particle size. The reasons I am sharing this is it's likely that eating the right fats (unprocessed) is not the problem!

When it comes to your heart health, here are the key players that you need to know about to understand your risk of heart disease:

— **Triglycerides:** these fats might be a better heart health indicator than LDL.

— **HDL:** the 'good' cholesterol that helps tidy up the LDL.

— **The triglyceride to HDL ratio:** a crucial indicator of heart disease risk.

The ratio is calculated by dividing your triglyceride by your HDL level. A lower ratio is ideal (less than 1.5) for a healthier balance and fewer small, dense LDL particles.

Remember that everyone's body is different. Some people are more sensitive to dietary fats due to genetics. If heart disease is in your family I recommend asking your doctor to do a blood test to look at your cholesterol mix.

The cholesterol story is more nuanced that we once thought. Focusing on whole foods, limiting refined carbs and sugars, and getting the right test can help you to be more resilient, but for personalised advice please consult a health professional.

I hope this provides some reassurance. While we're still learning, modern research has shed more light on the relationship between dietary fat and heart disease. The key takeaway is that sugar, refined carbs and trans fats (see below) may pose a greater risk than unprocessed fats from whole food sources.

Understanding different types of fats

Trans fats

These are the worst kind of fats for your health. They're man-made through a process called hydrogenation, which turns liquid vegetable oils into solid or semi-solid fats. You'll find trans fats in things like margarine, processed baked goods and fried foods. They increase your risk of heart disease, stroke and type 2 diabetes, so it's best to avoid them completely. While many countries have banned or limited their use, they can still be found in some processed foods, so always check the ingredients list for terms like trans fat, trans-unsaturated fatty acids, trans fatty acids, partially hydrogenated oils, partially hydrogenated vegetable oils, shortening and hardened fat.

Saturated fats

These fats come from animal products like meat, butter and cheese, as well as some plant sources like coconut oil. Your body actually makes all the saturated fat it needs, so you don't necessarily need to consume a lot from your diet.

While saturated fat has long been associated with increased cholesterol levels, particularly LDL cholesterol, recent research has shown that the relationship between saturated fat, cholesterol and health is more complex as previously discussed. This variability in response is due to genetic factors and overall metabolic health.

Some individuals may be more sensitive to dietary saturated fats than others, experiencing more pronounced increases in blood cholesterol levels in response to saturated fat intake. This individual variation highlights the complexity of the relationship between diet and health, and underscores the importance of personalised nutrition approaches.

Unsaturated fats

These are predominantly found in plant foods, such as vegetable oils, nuts and seeds, and fatty fish. These fats are considered helpful for improving cholesterol levels and reducing inflammation in the body. There are two types:

1. **Monounsaturated fats:** found in avocados, olives and olive oil, nuts, seeds and eggs.
2. **Polyunsaturated fats:** found in fatty fish (sardines, mackerel, herring, anchovies, salmon), walnuts, flaxseeds, chia seeds.

Within the polyunsaturated fats, are a crucial type called Essential Fatty Acids (EFAs) that your body can't produce on its own, so you need to get them from your diet. These are:

— **Omega-3s:** These include alpha-linolenic (ALA), found in plant sources like chia seeds and walnuts, as well as EPA and DHA (found in fatty fish and algae). DHA is particularly important for brain health, while EPA has anti-inflammatory effects.

— **Omega-6s:** The primary omega-6 is linoleic acid (LA), found in vegetable oils, nuts, seeds and grains. Your body can convert LA into another omega-6 called arachidonic acid (AA), which is also found in animal products.

These fats are crucial for the structure of all our cells — they make up the cell membranes and play a vital role in cellular function. They are also extremely important for brain health and cognitive function.

There are two specific fatty acids I want to highlight:

DHA (an omega-3): This is the primary structural component of cell membranes in your brain. It supports transmission of signals between nerve cells, influencing cognitive processes like learning and memory throughout your life. DHA also has neuroprotective properties, helping to safeguard brain cells from damage and resolving inflammation in the brain. Brain inflammation is linked to various neurological disorders, which can be contributed to by diets high in sugar and processed foods. It is the most important fat for your brain.

EPA (another omega-3): While not as concentrated in the brain as DHA, EPA plays a key role in modulating inflammation throughout the rest of your body. It has potent anti-inflammatory effects that help keep excessive inflammation at bay.

While you must eat these essential fatty acids, the key is to maintain a balance between omega-3s and omega-6s. Modern diets often have too many omega-6s and not enough omega-3s, which can contribute to inflammation.

Omega-3 fats are really the hero fats. Data points to their ability not only to protect you but to improve cognition, memory and focus.

Ok, so now you understand the different types of fats, what should you choose and how much?

The key is to ditch the 'fat fear' mindset and incorporate healthy fats into a balanced diet with adequate protein and fibre. When choosing to eat fats, your goal is to prioritise the fats the body needs and cannot make. Here is my recommended framework.

Start by removing all trans-fats (check labels) and refined vegetable oils — sunflower oil, rapeseed oil, safflower oil, corn oil, soybean oil, cottonseed oil, grapeseed oil. Just be aware that most restaurants use these vegetable oils, even fine-dining establishments. Then focus on the hero omega-3 fats, followed by mono-unsaturated fats from whole foods (from plants or animals).

Which fats to choose?

You want to include a source of healthy fats in most meals. I recommend that they make up approximately two thumb-sized portions per meal — you can eat one or two different options per meal. Some foods naturally contain healthy fats and protein together in nature, for example unprocessed animal foods like meat and cheese. However, meat is categorised as a protein source as it contains more protein than fat, while cheese is considered a fat source as it has a higher fat content.

This is just a guide to the amount of fats to consume; some people may want to increase this. Your aim is to get your plate balanced, choosing the right food initially, and you can increase the number of healthy fats to keep you satisfied and full once you are eating enough protein and fibre (see chapter 10).

1. Prioritise omega-3 fats from whole foods

— **Eat fatty fish**, such as sardines, salmon, herring, mackerel and anchovies 3–4 times per week (one serving counts as both your protein and fat source).

— **Eat omega-3 plant sources**, such as chia seeds, flaxseed and hemp seeds daily (1–2 tablespoons). If you are vegan or vegetarian it is particularly important to eat plant sources daily. Be aware that your body needs to convert plant sources of omega-3 into EPA and DHA and this conversion is limited, so I recommend supplementing with algae.

2. Choose mono-unsaturated fats from whole foods

— **Avocados** (¼–½ an avocado)

— **Olives** (6–10 olives per portion)

— **Raw nuts**, such as almonds, cashews, hazelnuts, pecans (one small handful per person)

— **Include extra virgin olive oil daily:**
    — Choose cold-pressed and unrefined.
    — Use 2 tablespoons per day; I encourage my clients to add it raw by drizzling it over cooked food.
    — Heat to no more than 185 degrees. For cooking at high heat use avocado oil or coconut oil, which have higher smoking points.

Note: *Cooking at high temperatures can make oils go rancid. This happens when the oil breaks down and*

*forms harmful compounds, like aldehydes, which create
unpleasant flavours and odours. The nutritional value
of the oil can also degrade.*

3. Saturated fats

When choosing saturated fat from meat, remember to
buy the best-quality meat you can — ideally organic and
grass-fed — knowing that the animal is eating appropriate
food for their species. (Eggs, meat and Greek yoghurt are
considered proteins and are discussed in the protein chapter).

What about eggs?

I know what you are probably thinking — do I need to
worry about the number of eggs I can eat for cholesterol?
This question comes up a lot in my clinic. Eggs are a highly
nutritious food. They contain rich sources of vitamin A,
B12 and choline, the precursor to one of the brain's main
neurotransmitters — acetylcholine, which is crucial for
your memory and learning. They are also a good source
of protein and easy to cook — I like to refer to them as
nature's fast food. I encourage my clients to eat 2–3 eggs
daily because they are so nutrient-dense. Several studies
have shown no link between egg consumption and heart
disease when eating a balanced diet. According to
Dr Georgia Ede, if you add 3 eggs per day to people's usual
diets for weeks in a row, in most cases, their cholesterol
won't move. About one-third of subjects will see a slight
raise in LDL-C but also see a rise in HDL-C, so their overall
ratio doesn't change.

What about dairy?

Dairy products can contain high-quality protein that provides all the essential amino acids, making dairy a good choice for vegetarians. Dairy products can cause some people digestive issues, acne and eczema, to name a few, and this may be linked to an allergy or an intolerance. Dairy also contains a carbohydrate, primarily in the form of lactose, a naturally-occurring sugar that doesn't spike blood sugar levels as rapidly as refined sugars do. The presence of other components in dairy can help to slow the glucose response.

If you eat dairy, choose full-fat, ideally grass-fed products as they are more satisfying and the least processed (check labels). Fermented dairy can be easier to digest and contains beneficial bacteria that contribute to gut health.

A great way to incorporate healthy fats into your food is to see them as a flavour enhancer. They can add richness and texture to your dishes. Here are some ideas:

Nuts and seeds

Mix together a variety of raw nuts and seeds — hemp seed hearts, pumpkin seeds, sunflower seeds, hazelnuts, almonds, pecans, cashews and walnuts and store in a large reusable jar, then:

— Chop them up and sprinkle over meat, fish and/or vegetables.

— Use a pestle and mortar to grind them down to make a nut and seed 'breadcrumb' to sprinkle over proteins and/or vegetables.

— Try making nutty bean dips, blending white beans, nuts, olive oil, garlic and lemon.

— Experiment with tahini: it makes a beautiful rich and tasty dressing when blended with garlic, mustard, lemon juice and water.

— Toast batches of nuts in a dry frying pan and store in a reusable jar.

Olive oil

— Drizzle over salads to bring them alive (they are also rich in polyphenols — more on this in chapter 11).

— Make a simple olive oil dressing with raw garlic and balsamic or apple cider vinegar (see page 116).

Cheese

— Crumble goat's cheese or feta over trays of roasted vegetables.

— Shave parmesan over salads.

— Add a little feta to scrambled eggs with spinach.

Avocado and olives

— Enjoy avocado mashed on toast, in smoothies and salads.

— Make a homemade guacamole with white beans and a little chilli, olive oil and lemon juice.

— Add olives to your salad.

You can see how easily healthy fats can really change your food and bring excitement to your plate — just remember these ideas and get used to practising them.

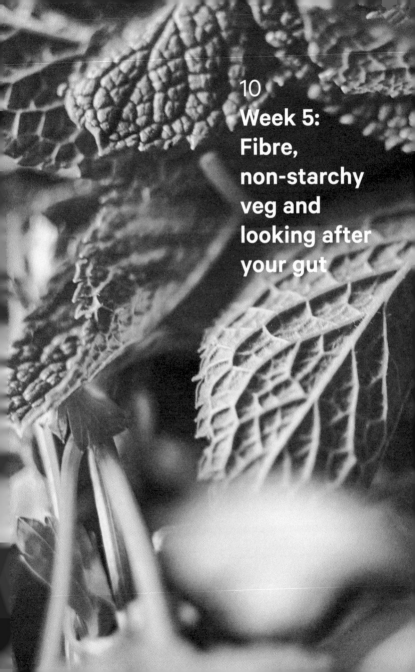

10

Week 5: Fibre, non-starchy veg and looking after your gut

We all know vegetables are good for us. But what if their benefits go far beyond just vitamins and minerals?

In this chapter, I will show you just how good they are, sharing the many roles they serve in keeping your body running smoothly, supporting metabolic health and modifying your immunity and mind, which means that they can adjust and influence your immune system and cognitive function, therefore enhancing your overall health resilience.

Let's begin by talking about the fibre found in vegetables and plant foods — another ally for feeling full and balanced. For years, fibre might have been on your radar as the stuff in wholemeal bread — something you eat for regularity's sake. Fibre is so much more than that. Fibre is magic and has a crucial role your overall health.

What is fibre?

Fibre is part of a carbohydrate you cannot fully digest and acts differently to carbs inside your body. The higher the fibre content in a food with carbs, the less of an impact the carbs have on your blood sugar and the more beneficial they are for your overall health.

There are two main types of fibre: soluble and insoluble — both play a critical role in health by forming a gel on the inside of the gut that slows down your digestion, therefore reducing the rate at which sugar and starches reach your bloodstream. This gives your insulin time to do its job, keeping blood sugar levels stable and preventing unwanted spikes. Fibre also triggers the release of satiety hormones, chemical messengers that tell your brain, 'Hey, I'm feeling full.' This reduces cravings and helps you avoid overeating, which can overload your system.

Studies have consistently shown that people who enjoyed more fibre-rich vegetables had a lower risk of developing insulin resistance, suggesting a high-fibre diet can reduce the risk by 20–30 per cent.

This is one of the major problems with the processed food industry — it's not only what's been added to the food, but also what's been removed — fibre!

Fibre also plays a vital role in protecting your body's fortress – your gut. Your gut is super important. We don't fully understand how it works yet, but we know how vital it is to health, so you need to nurture and look after it.

When healthy, your gut protects you from allergies, improves your nutritional status, regulates your metabolism, improves glucose control and insulin sensitivity and supports your mitochondria (cells that are responsible for generating energy) as well as helping to regulate your mood. Your gut helps you to keep inflammation at bay when nourished and working well.

Imagine your gut as a castle, protecting your body from invaders. The key to its strength lies in the tiniest of allies: your gut bacteria. These bacteria work in unison with us to promote health; however when they are not in balance, they may initiate disease. These little warriors thrive on dietary fibre. They need you!

Your gut is a tightly woven net made up of epithelial cells, forming an inner wall. This net structure acts as a guard stopping anything harmful from sneaking into your bloodstream. Protecting these cells is another layer of defense, a sticky shield of mucus. This precious shield is crafted by your very own gut bacteria, fuelled by the fibre you eat. When you eat a good amount of fibre, this feeds them and so they build a thick and stronger shield, keeping your gut lining safe and sound and ultimately making your entire immune system a tight fortress. You feed them; they protect you. It's a beautiful partnership.

But that's not all. These good gut bacteria can also produce molecules that send signals up to your brain. They can tell your brain that you're full and satisfied, helping curb cravings.

One special resident among your gut bacteria that is getting a lot of attention is Akkermansia, a friendly bacterium that plays a key role in metabolic health. A low presence in the gut has been associated with obesity, inflammation, diabetes, anxiety, depression, gut barrier dysfunction, neurological disorders and metabolic dysfunction. Think of it like a tiny insulin assistant. Akkermansia produces beneficial compounds that further cool down inflammation and even creates short-chain fatty acids that may directly improve how your cells respond to insulin.

So, by incorporating fibre-rich foods you're not just supporting Akkermansia, you're investing in a healthier, smoother-running metabolism. The problem is you are likely not eating enough fibre! It seems that less than 10 per cent of most western populations consume adequate levels of dietary fibre, with typical consumption being at about half the recommended levels.

The recommended daily fibre intake is approximately 30 grams per day for men and 25 grams per day for women. In the UK studies suggest the average intake is approximately 15 grams, the intake across the US is similar. Low fibre intake may mean that your gut allies are underfed and if they are underfed they can begin to feed on your sticky shield of mucin, reducing your defense.

Fermented foods

One way to support your gut bacteria is to eat fermented foods, also known as probiotic foods. These foods contain live microorganisms that colonise in your gut to maintain a healthy balance of friendly bacteria, so eating fermented foods daily is important. Research has shown that consuming six servings of fermented foods per day increased microbiome diversity and improved immune responses in healthy adults. A serving is approximately 2–4 tablespoons of kimchi or sauerkraut, and approximately 150ml of yoghurt or kefir. Six sounds like a lot, but you can begin by adding a little to every meal and building up. If you have never eaten fermented foods before, start by eating one each day. Sauerkraut, kimchi, live probiotic yoghurt, pickled vegetables, kefir, kombucha, kimchi, miso, fermented soy (natto and tempeh) are all great choices. When introducing fermented foods it is important to do so slowly, increasing the quantity you consume gradually. Start with a small amount, such as 1 tablespoon of kimchi or sauerkraut, and increase that over time. This allows your gut to adjust to the probiotic-rich food. If you have a sensitive gut it is recommended that you start with 1 teaspoon.

Micronutrients

As well as providing a good source of fibre, vegetables boast an abundance of micronutrients that play critical roles in proper bodily functioning and disease prevention.

Micronutrient deficiencies have far-reaching impacts on the body. Lacking vitamins like C, zinc and iron weakens your immune system, leaving you more susceptible to illnesses. B vitamins, iodine and folate are crucial for brain health — deficiencies can impair cognition, neurotransmitters and mental wellbeing. Hormonal imbalances can arise from lacking iodine, zinc and selenium, which regulate hormone production. Micronutrients are mighty important.

In the US and UK, many adults suffer from deficiencies in key micronutrients, including low folate levels. But folate isn't the only culprit. Deficiencies in magnesium, vitamin D, zinc and vitamin B12 occur in both countries. These micronutrient deficiencies have been linked to an increased risk of type 2 diabetes and can impair its management.

When I run blood tests in my clinic, so many of my clients have below optimal levels of B12, folate, zinc and D. I recommend that you have these markers checked to make sure they are optimal. If you are vegan, you must absolutely supplement with B12. All of us should be taking vitamin D over the autumn, winter and spring. To supplement the appropriate levels of vitamin D it's important to know your blood vitamin D level. You can consult a practitioner who can help you to identity low nutrient levels. There are also a number of direct-to-consumer testing labs that you can use (see page 140).

All these micronutrients play crucial roles in insulin action, reducing oxidative stress, controlling inflammation and supporting your nervous system — all vital for maintaining healthy blood sugar levels and these are just a few examples.

There is, however, a crucial gap between the minimum amount of a nutrient needed to prevent deficiency and the optimal amount for optimal health and wellbeing.

Your individual needs for micronutrients can vary based on your health status, your age, life load (everything in your day-to-day that demands your time, energy and attention) and genetics. You will likely need more than the RDA (recommended daily allowance) as this is focused on preventing disease rather than achieving optimal health. The more you can obtain through food the better.

Research also shows a clear link between increased fruit and vegetable consumption and greater happiness, less stress and better overall mood! In one trial, young adults who received daily fruit and vegetable boxes felt significantly more energised, motivated and fulfilled. While the reasons aren't fully understood, the evidence is mounting — incorporating more greens, reds and oranges into your diet could be an easy, natural path to elevated wellbeing.

Your goal this week is to feed your gut, fire up your mitochondria and nurture your cells by loading up on top fibre foods that are packed with micronutrients, namely, non-starchy vegetables. So don't be shy about piling them high on your plate. Your happier self will thank you.

So, what are non-starchy veg and how much should you eat?

— **Cruciferous veg:** broccoli, kale, cauliflower, cabbage (red and white), radish, chard, rocket, brussel sprouts, bok choy/pak choi

— **Dark leafy greens:** spinach, Swiss chard and watercress

- **Sulphur-loving foods:** onions (red and white), garlic and leeks

- **Other veg:** peppers, courgettes, mushrooms, celery, cucumber, aubergine, tomatoes, green beans, lettuce, artichoke and chicory

Non-starchy veg contain the ideal, balanced carb-to-fibre ratio. You calculate the ratio by dividing the total carbs by the grams of fibre and it gives you an assessment of the quality of carbohydrates in your food. Generally a 5:1 ratio is considered ideal for supporting blood sugar. This means that for every 5 grams of carbs, there should be 1 gram of fibre. This is a general guideline and not a strict rule, though many non-starchy vegetables conform to this. By simply eating half a plate of non-starchy vegetables with both lunch and dinner you can easily boost your fibre and micronutrient intake.

The healthiest non-starchy veg are the dark leafy greens and cruciferous veg because they are the most nutrient-dense and the most powerful when it comes to protecting your brain. Cruciferous veggies contain a fascinating compound called sulforaphane. This natural wonder can actually activate your body's own antioxidant defenses by flipping on a 'master switch' gene. This tells your cells to increase the production of powerful antioxidant enzymes and detoxifying proteins. It's like giving your internal defence system a big boost, helping to neutralise harmful free radicals and keep you healthier from the inside out.

Here's a basic framework to help you eat more non-starchy vegetables:

1. Start by making sure you have vegetables incorporated into both lunch and dinner. An easy way to do this is by adding a green side salad or some raw veggie sticks like carrot, cucumber, peppers, celery with a tasty hummus or yoghurt dip.

2. Make those vegetables taste amazing with different spices, herbs and dressings (see pages 122–125).

3. Now take a look at your typical lunch and dinner plates. Is half of your plate dedicated to non-starchy vegetables? If not, that is the goal to work towards by increasing the amounts slowly.

4. If you are already managing to get vegetables in both meals, try increasing the portions gradually. Add an extra helping of your usual vegetables to get closer to that half a plate goal.

5. Once you are eating half a plate, you can start exploring a wider variety of different non-starchy veg options.

6. Remember to incorporate fermented food. Start with adding them to one meal a day, then increase this to every meal. Top savoury dishes with sauerkraut, eat fermented yoghurt or kefir with breakfast and enjoy a low-sugar kombucha drink. Use miso to flavour food and dressings.

7. Remember to prioritise leafy greens and cruciferous veg. You can then begin to assess colour and diversity —the more colour on your plate the better as colour provides a diverse range of polyphenols (see page 113).

Tips for eating more non-starchy vegetables:

— Stir spinach into scrambled eggs or tofu.

— Add a leafy green to your morning smoothie.

— Add grated or chopped veggies to your favourite soups, stews, curries and sauces.

— Make a tray of roasted vegetables with enough to eat cold the next day.

— Choose to eat stir-fries weekly — they are an easy and quick way to eat more veg (see page 126).

— Eat salads for lunch — they don't have to be boring.

— Swap rice for cauliflower rice or broccoli rice.

— Swap pasta for cabbage strips or courgette spirals.

— Make a homemade coleslaw that last up to 4 days and serve with each meal (this is one of my favourite things to do; see page 149).

— Have frozen veg in the freezer.

— As a back up, take pre-washed salad bags to work or have them in your fridge during times when your diary is looking busy.

— Prep veg in advance. Wash, chop and store veg in containers ready for use in the week (remember, where possible aim to cook once a day, and to prep two meals at this time so you have another meal ready for the next day).

11

Week 6: Polyphenols and spicing up your plate

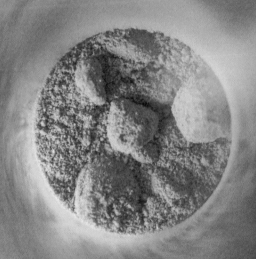

We've all been there, staring blankly into the fridge, completely uninspired about what to make for dinner... again. Cooking can sometimes feel monotonous, with the same familiar flavours and dishes on rotation. Clients often tell me they get bored with their food.

But what if I told you that there's an easy way to spice up your meals and achieve health benefits at the same time. I often tell my clients that when it comes to diversity, it's about creating simple dressings and sauces using herbs and spices. You will mostly likely have a shortlist of your typical proteins, carbs and veggies you enjoy. The real potential for making them interesting is found in your spice cabinet.

This chapter is about simple ways to add flavour and excitement so you can fall back in love with your food.

At home you probably have a host of spices and herbs that you may use from time to time when you are following a recipe. I suspect the rest of the time they sit in your cupboard. You don't need to be a chef to create great flavour combinations, it's about experimenting a little and being creative in your kitchen.

Deanna Minich refers to herbs and spices as 'The Many Medicines Cabinet'. I love this and I want you to think of your spice cupboard as your 'Flavours Cabinet'. Every time you make your food, I want you to ask yourself, how am I going to amplify this dish? I will show you how, but first, I want to share the power these foods bring to your health.

Meet the polyphenol

Polyphenols are like magical components found in many foods and drinks that do wonders for your body. They are a diverse group of natural compounds found in plants; they also form the pigments that lend vibrant colours to spices, herbs, fruits, vegetables, nuts, seeds and even beverages like tea and coffee. They are part of a plant's immune system, helping plants stay healthy by boosting its tolerance and nutrient uptake to thrive in its environment. Your immune system also benefits from these properties when you eat them. These bioactive compounds act as antioxidants, shielding your cells from harmful free radicals and chronic disease and fighting off damage from things like inflammation and oxidative stress and reducing the risk of getting an infection.

Even more exciting is their role in modifying your genes. Polyphenols may actually help make your cells stronger and more resilient through a process called 'hormesis', which induces positive stress on the body. While you may have heard of this concept in the context of exercise — where the stress of physical activity makes your body stronger; it's intriguing to note that plants elicit a similar response. Plants contain trace amounts of these chemicles, which act like a mild stressor when we eat them. This can potentially influence how your genes are turned on or off, helping your body's natural defences. By consuming plants, you're harnessing the power of positive stress for biological resilience.

We know that these foods taste amazing, but what's truly surprising is that polyphenols directly interact with proteins in your saliva to modify and enhance the flavours you experience, amplifying your sensory enjoyment of meals in an unexpected way.

The majority of nutrients, including carbohydrates, proteins and fats, are digested in the small intestine. Polyphenols, however, are not fully absorbed in the small intestine. They make their way to your colon (large intestine), where they interact with the bacteria living in your gut and help the good bacteria to grow and thrive. We are learning that the more diverse these bacteria the healthier and more resilient you are. Think of a forest: the more plants and species, the greater the ecosystem's health and richness. This is also true for your gut microbiome.

Polyphenols can also directly protect your brain cells from damage as their antioxidant properties can shield them from stress. And evidence suggests they may help promote the formation of new connections between brain cells, potentially helping delay the onset of neurodegenerative diseases, such as Alzheimer's or Parkinson's. There's also evidence that they may help balance out your mood by influencing feel-good brain chemicals like serotonin and dopamine. Berry polyphenols (anthocyanins) which are particularly enriched in wild blueberries have shown potential effects both directly in the brain, as well as improving the health of the gut and cardiovascular system at doses of 1–2 cups of blueberries per day. The science is still emerging, but there's definitely a lot of exciting potential when it comes to the benefits of polyphenols.

There are over 8,000 types of polyphenol and they can be divided into four primary categories that include the majority: flavonoids, phenolic acid, lignans and stilbenes. Spices tend to be higher in polyphenols on a gram per gram level than other foods.

The best foods for polyphenols

— **Berries,** such as blackberries, elderberries, blueberries, strawberries and raspberries.

— **Other fruit:** pomegranate, blackcurrants, apples, plums.

— **Cocoa:** cocoa powder and dark chocolate (minimum of 85 per cent cocoa solids).

— **Coffee and tea** (both black and green tea).

— **Spices and herbs:** cloves, peppermint, star anise, sage, rosemary, thyme, ginger and cinnamon.

— **Nuts and seeds:** hazelnuts, walnuts, almonds, pecans, flaxseeds and sesame seeds.

— **Vegetables:** artichokes, red and green chicory, red and white onions, spinach, broccoli, carrots, asparagus.

— **Legumes:** black beans, red kidney beans, pinto beans and white beans.

— **Olives and olive oil.**

Experiment with eating as many polyphenol-rich foods as you can. I am going to share five simple and quick ways to elevate your food and your enjoyment. There's no need to buy shop-bought condiments, sauces and dressings which often contain troublesome ingredients and chemicals.

1. Salad dressings

Ask any of my friends, and they'll tell you — I'm utterly devoted to salads. No matter the season, I find salads are the perfect way for combining all the pillars of nourishment into one amazing flavoursome meal. A good salad is all about the dressing.

Salad dressings are quick and easy and you can invent endless combinations in no time. Below is a basic formula you can use. You can make dressings in bulk and store them in a jar in the fridge for up to a week for quick easy use.

Method:

— Choose your ingredients following the basic formula: acid + oil + emulsifier + flavour and texture.

— Combine all the ingredients in a bowl or jar and whisk/shake.

— Experiment with the flavour and texture element — add more than one to your dressing.

— Season to your taste with salt and pepper.

— Dress the salad when it is ready to eat.

— You can serve extra dressing on the side.

1 part acid

1 tablespoon

Apple cider vinegar

Balsamic vinegar

Lemon juice

Lime

Red wine vinegar

3 parts oil

3 tablespoons

Extra virgin olive oil

Tahini (2 parts mixed with
1 part water)

Avocado oil

1 emulsifier

1 teaspoon

English mustard

Dijon mustard

Wholegrain mustard

Flavour and texture

*to your taste — you can combine
more than one*

Almond butter

Avocado

Coconut yoghurt

Full-fat Greek yoghurt

Honey

Miso

Olives

Peanut butter

Spring onion

Red onion

Tahini

Dried herbs/spices:

Basil

Capers

Chilli flakes

Cumin seeds

Fennel seeds

Ginger (crushed or grated)

Oregano

Thyme

Turmeric

Soy sauce

Sumac

Za'atar

2. Pesto

I usually recommend using dried herbs and spices in salad dressings and fresh herbs in pesto.

To make a pesto you will need a blender, grinder or a pestle and mortar. Follow a similar formula to this one:

— 100–150ml extra virgin olive oil (for a runny pesto)

— 1–2 handfuls of fresh herbs (any will do)

— 1 garlic clove (optional)

— 1–3 tablespoons of nuts or seeds of your choice (optional)

— 1–2 tablespoons of acid (see table opposite)

Method:

— Choose a combination of fresh herbs.

— Blend or grind everything together.

— Season with salt and pepper to taste.

— Store in an airtight container in the fridge, covered with a layer of oil to preserve them.

— Use within 5–7 days.

Acid

1–2 tablespoons

Apple cider vinegar
Balsamic vinegar
Lemon juice
Lime juice
Red wine vinegar

Oil

100–150ml extra virgin olive oil

Extra virgin olive oil
Avocado (if using use less olive oil)

Garlic

1 clove, optional

Nuts or seeds

1–3 tablespoons, optional

Fresh herbs

*1–2 handfuls of fresh herbs
— you can use a single herb or
use a mix of up to three*

Basil
Dill
Chives
Coriander
Marjoram
Mint
Oregano
Parsley
Rosemary
Sage
Tarragon
Thyme

*Option to add a dried herb or spice
too to boost the polyphenols —
1 teaspoon (see list above)*

Feel free to experiment with the ratios based on your taste preference. Increase the herb quantity if you want a stronger herb flavour. Adjust the oil and nuts and seeds to suit your texture preference. You can also add a hard cheese, such as parmesan.

Serve 1–2 tablespoons with food, add to fish, meat, beans, vegetables, dips or use as a salad dressing. Some pesto combinations I like include:

— Basil, oregano, rosemary and thyme

— Coriander and pumpkin seeds

— Dill and avocado

— Mint, dill and chives

— Rocket and walnuts

— Parsley and pine nuts

— Parsley, basil and thyme

— Parsley, chives and tarragon

— Parsley, mint and capers

— Thyme and oregano

— Oregano and parsley

3. Marinades, rubs and seasoning

Marinades and rubs

Marinating proteins or vegetables is another great way to infuse them with flavour. Combine your chosen spice blend with olive oil and acidic ingredients like lemon juice or vinegar; you can add garlic and ginger too. You can also make a dry rub by mixing the spice blend with salt, pepper and other dry seasonings. Coat proteins or vegetables in this rub before cooking.

Don't be afraid to try new combinations and discover your own signature flavour profiles. Most spices are fat-soluble, so use in combination with oils. Toasting whole spices like cloves, coriander seeds or cumin seeds in a dry pan over a low heat before grinding releases their full aromatic potential.

On the next page there is a table you can use to create your own pairings and blends.

Pepper pot seasoning

I often ask my clients to do this as it's so simple. Get a pepper pot and fill it with a combination of dried spices. Place on your kitchen table. Every time you eat, season your food with spices, black pepper and a good mineral salt.

Spice	Pair with	Food partners
Cacao	*Sweet spices:* vanilla, cinnamon, liquorice. *Savoury spices:* chilli, bay, ginger, coriander.	Add to smoothies, yoghurt. Cacao nibs (nutty crunchy texture) — sprinkle over fruit salads, yoghurts, or add to banana bread, flapjacks, homemade cookies.
Chilli	Ginger, turmeric, lemongrass, cumin, coriander, cardamom, black pepper, mustard, Sichuan pepper.	Use to add heat to dishes, as well as flavour. Sprinkle over a tomato salad. Add to a tomato-based sauce. Combine with others spices to make a stir-fry sauce and curries. Use in a dry marinade for proteins.
Cinnamon	*For savoury dishes:* allspice, cumin, peppercorn, cardamom. *For sweet dishes:* nutmeg, cacao and cardamon.	Scatter ground cinnamon over fruit and add to smoothies. Add to banana bread, flapjacks and other bakes. Add to yoghurts and hot chocolate. Add a stick to stews, curries or a noodle broth.
Coriander	Cardamon, cumin, nutmeg, black pepper, ginger, lemongrass.	Toss the whole seeds in homemade coleslaws — using raw veg like cabbage, celery carrots etc. Use ground in a dry marinade for proteins. Add to pulses and lentils.

Spice	Pair with	Food partners
Cumin	Black pepper, cinnamon, cardamom, coriander, nigella, star anise.	Toast whole, crush seeds and sprinkle on root vegetables, carrots, parsnips, beetroot, sweet potatoes. Add to pulses and other lentils. Scatter over hummus. Use ground in a rub for meats. Combine ground with lemon and yoghurt to make a dressing for salads and vegetables. Use ground in a dry marinade for proteins.
Fennel	Enhances sweet and savoury dishes. *Sweet spices:* nutmeg, star anise. *Savoury spices:* black pepper, cumin. Build citrus notes with cardamom.	Add toasted to fruits. Add to chutneys. Sprinkle into homemade nut and seed trail mix. Add to vegetables and lentil stews. Mix with other spices to create protein rubs. Crush seeds over fish.
Garlic	Works as a trio with onions and ginger. Pair with all herbs and spices. Garlic amplifies and brings other flavours together.	Chop and crush before using and allow the garlic to stand for 10 minutes — this helps the bioactive ingredient allicin to fully develop.[1] Use more than one clove in cooking. Add raw to salad dressings, pestos, dips, marinades, sauces and rubs.

---

1   Allicin is a compound that has antimicrobial, antioxidant and anti-inflammatory
     effects. It supports the immune system and may even help with cardiovascular
     health and blood sugar regulation. When you chop and allow the garlic to stand
     for 10 minutes this beneficial compound can develop.

Spice	Pair with	Food partners
Ginger	*For savoury dishes:* chilli, black pepper, to build heat. Lemongrass and coriander for citrus flavours. *For sweet dishes:* cinnamon, nutmeg and cacao.	Add fresh or dried to hot water and lemon. Use to make a stir-fry sauce. Great with fish. Add grated to Asian-style coleslaws. Use ground ginger in baking.
Oregano	Basil, parsley, sage, mint, thyme, rosemary, coriander.	Add to tomato-based sauces. Use fresh to make pestos. Use dried to make rubs for fish, chicken, tofu and vegetables. Add dried to a salad dressing.
Paprika	*Savoury spices:* cardamon, coriander, ginger, oregano, thyme. *Sweet spices:* cacao, allspice, cinnamon, ginger.	Sprinkle over hummus and dips. Add to marinades and rubs for protein and vegetables. Use in Mediterranean-style dishes and combine with herbs.
Rosemary	Thyme, oregano, marjoram, basil, black pepper, sage.	Roast with vegetables and meats. Add to hot water with a little lemon to make a drink. Use to make a pesto.
Thyme	Basil, parsley, sage, chives, coriander, mint.	Roast with vegetables. Use in marinades and pestos

Spice	Pair with	Food partners
Turmeric	*Savoury spices:* cumin, paprika, cardamom, black pepper. *Sweet spices:* cardamom, ginger. *For sweet dishes:* cinnamon, nutmeg and cacao.	Use to make drinks with warm milk, ginger, a little raw honey and black pepper (this increases bioavailability). Add to hot water with a little lemon, fresh ginger and black pepper. Add to curry dishes, stews and rubs for proteins and vegetables. Sprinkle over dips.

Dried spice blend combinations

Typically 1–2 teaspoons per spice to make the blend.
Keep the more pungent spices to ¼ teaspoon, for example chilli, cardamom, cayenne pepper, star anise and cloves:

— **Garam masala:** cloves, cinnamon, cardamon and black pepper.

— **Curry powder:** turmeric, coriander, cumin and chilli.

— **Cajun:** paprika, garlic powder, onion powder, black pepper, cayenne pepper and sometimes thyme.

— **Chinese five spice blend:** star anise, cinnamon, cloves, Sichuan peppercorns and fennel seeds.

— **Mediterranean:** sage, rosemary, thyme, marjoram and sometimes paprika.

4. Stir-fry sauces

A stir-fry is a quick and versatile meal and a great way to eat more veg varieties and include spices. It only takes around 10 minutes to make once you have chopped your veg. Add a little water to the olive oil, if you are using that as your cooking oil, to keep the temperature down; alternatively use coconut oil. You want to cook your vegetables quickly to keep their crunch and preserve the nutrients.

Method:

— Choose one item from each section below.

— Place all the ingredients in a bowl or jar and mix.

— The sauces can also be used as marinades for your proteins.

Salt	Oil	Sweet
2 tablespoons	*2–3 tablespoons*	*1 teaspoon, optional*
Tamari	Olive oil	Honey
Soy sauce	Avocado oil	Molasses
Miso		Maple Syrup

Acid	Spice/herb	Seeds
1–2 tablespoons	*1 teaspoon*	*1 tablespoon*
Lemon	Garlic	Sesame seeds
Lime	Chill	Sunflower seeds
	Ginger	Pumpkin seeds
	Coriander	Peanuts
	Cumin	

5. Drinks

You can also drink your polyphenols:

— To your coffee add ground cinnamon, ginger and turmeric. Or swap your coffee to a turmeric latte.

— To smoothies add ground cinnamon, ginger or turmeric.

I hope you are feeling as excited as me about bringing more flavour to your food. You can choose the same proteins, vegetables and carbs each week and completely shift their taste experience using spices and herbs. Polyphenols make your food taste better and do wonders for your health!

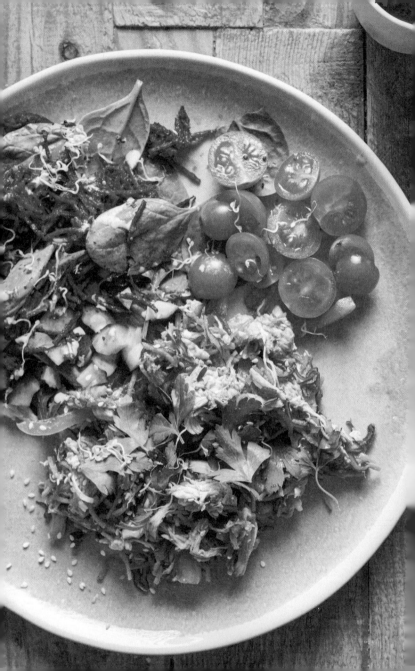

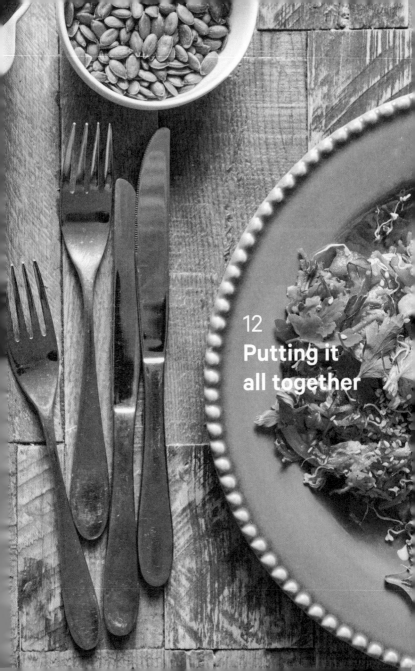

12
Putting it all together

That's been one of my mantras — focus and simplicity. Simple can be harder than complex: You have to work hard to get your thinking clean to make it simple. But it's worth it in the end because once you get there, you can move mountains.

Steve Jobs

The health and wellness industry can make us think optimal health and nutrition is complicated.

Information overload drowns out your own innate wisdom about what feels good for your body. It can fuel insecurities and suck the joy right out of food. You stop celebrating your amazingly unique self and lose touch with how to truly nourish your body from the inside out.

At the same time, our conventional medical system's tendency to treat symptoms and body parts in isolation — the gastroenterologist for your gut, cardiologist for your heart, dermatologist for skin, neurologist for brain — is disconnected and frequently misses the underlying causes of a problem, which are often tied to lifestyle and nutrition.

But here's what I always tell my clients: symptoms are simply messages, not to be silenced but listened to. You must look inward and explore where imbalances may exist. Conventional medicine teaches us to slap a plaster over the symptom and often ignores its causes.

Most of the adjustments needed to live better, build resilience and address imbalances — quality sleep, movement, stress management, social connection — don't cost a thing; you just need to invest in nourishing yourself.

The human body is admittedly complex, but the solutions for thriving are simple at their core. I appreciate you sticking with me through the scientific explanations, which provide important context. But the answers remain refreshingly straightforward. You already have an innate intuition about how to feed yourself well. When you clear away the clutter and outside noise, you can listen to your body's signals and trust yourself to make the right choices.

More recently, advancements have enhanced our ability to understand and support our health. Thanks to improved access to testing and wearable devices, we now have more opportunity than ever before to gain deeper insights into our personal physiology and specific needs. This combination of intuitive wisdom and technological support empowers us to make informed decisions.

You now know what to do and what every meal needs to look like to eat for resilience, so to recap, here are my core principles for feeling your best, most nourished self:

1. **Ignore diets; they don't work, think about nourishment instead.**

2. **Good nutrition is about feeding the body what it needs and cannot make. Ask yourself, how do you want to feel, not what do you want to eat.**

3. **The food you eat builds you and your cells and determines how well you function.**

4. **When you eat this way, you feel full, satisfied and nourished and you will thrive.**

5. **Be filled with the incredible power of real, unprocessed food.**

6. **Fall back in love with food.**

Now, I'd love you to complete the table opposite. This is your personalised nutrition plan; you can refer back to this table weekly. You don't need to rely on recipes to know how to eat, just keep referring back to chapter 11 to inspire new and different flavour combinations.

In every column list your favourite foods for each category. Once you have done this, when thinking about what to eat simply choose one item from each column.

Welcome to your perfect nutrition plan!

Lastly, refer to the traffic light system in chapter 3 (see page 48). Redo the activity a second time and see how far you have come. Remember this is your tool to check in with where you are at, or if you feel like things have slipped to help guide you back to nourishment. Remember life will always get in the way, and things won't go to plan, and that's okay. Strength and resilience come from getting back to plan as quickly as you can. And when you do, you'll be stronger.

And finally remember this important perspective on food choices: instead of asking yourself, 'What do I want to eat?', ask 'How do I want to feel?'. This helps change your perspective on your choices. You have the power to nourish your body and mind through the foods you consume. Food is your opportunity to build resilience, energy and vitality every day.

Your personalised nutrition plan

Proteins	Non-starchy veg	Healthy fats	Complex carbs	Spices	Fermented foods
1–2 palm-sized portions (prioritise omega-3s)	*½ a plate*	*1–2 thumb-sized portions (prioritise omega-3s)*	*1 cupped handful*		

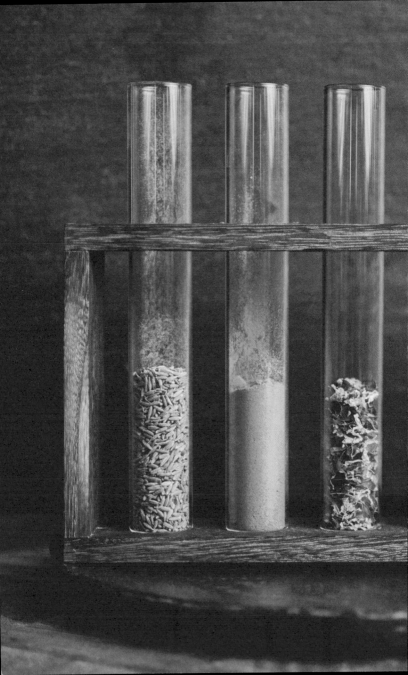

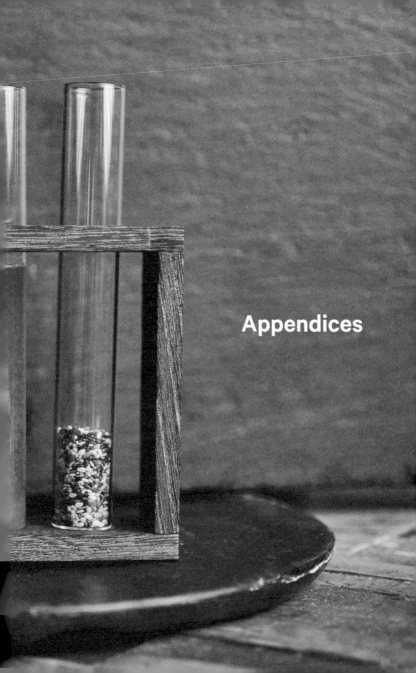
Appendices

Testing

I encourage all my clients to know their baseline metabolic markers and I would advise you to do the same. Knowing these numbers can be a good way for you to take control and responsibility for tracking your health, in addition to having annual blood tests. These blood markers tell you how well your body is producing energy and how well that energy is entering your cells and enabling them to function.

Opposite is a list of the blood tests that you can mostly access through your family doctor to provide you with these markers. Understanding the markers is crucial because so often I see clients dismiss niggling symptoms, even referring to them as, 'just normal for me'. However, symptoms like persistent fatigue, digestive issues, anxiety, skin issues or PMS symptoms like low mood or painful cramps are not normal. They can often be indicators for underlying imbalances that blood tests can help identify.

It is important to understand that outward appearance is not an accurate indicator of internal health. You can look perfectly healthy on the outside and have imbalanced blood sugar levels or other hidden elevated markers. Many modern-day diseases can start silently, often without obvious symptoms in the early stages.

My aim with my clients is to uncover their current health status and reduce future risk. This should be your goal too. By knowing your blood markers you gain valuable insights into your body's internal functioning, allowing you to take proactive steps towards optimal health. Your healthcare provider or nutritionist will guide you with specific actions to take to address any imbalances or suboptimal markers. Typical blood markers you can ask your family doctor to run include:

Marker	Unit	What is this	What your number means
Triglycerides (TG)	mmol/L	A type of fat very much influenced by dietary consumption. Responsible for storing extra calories.	Elevated levels can indicate poor control of blood sugar.
Fasting glucose	mmol/L	Snapshot of the amount of sugar present in the blood. Has a direct effect on energy levels.	Increased blood sugar is associated with type 1 and 2 diabetes, metabolic syndrome and high insulin.
HBA1C	mmol/L	Average blood sugar over the last 3 months.	Increased levels are associated with insulin resistance and diabetes.
Cholesterol LDL-C	mmol/L	Considered the 'bad' cholesterol, it transports cholesterol and other fatty acids from the liver to peripheral tissues.	An increased level is just one of many independent risk factors for cardiovascular disease.

Marker	Unit	What is this	What your number means
Cholesterol HDL-C	mmol/L	Transports cholesterol from peripheral tissues back to the liver for processing and metabolising. This process is thought to be protective against atherosclerosis (a build up of plaque in the arteries) and heart disease.	A low level is thought to accelerate the development of atherosclerosis and is a risk factor for heart disease.
Liver enzymes ALT, GGT, AST		Liver enzymes that are released during liver damage.	Higher than optimal levels can indicate a sluggish liver and show if damage has occurred.
C-Reactive Protein	mg/L	General marker of inflammation.	When elevated it is a sign of low-grade inflammation.
Vitamin D	nmol/L	Fat-soluble vitamin synthesised from the skin.	Low levels are associated with many disorders including hypertension, diabetes, cardiovascular disease, chronic inflammation, pain, low mood, diabetes and autoimmunity.
Vitamin B12	pg/ml	A water-soluble vitamin critical for growth and repair, the brain, cardiovascular health, metabolic health, mood and energy.	A deficiency can cause neurological symptoms, fatigue and a particular type of anaemia.

Marker	Unit	What is this	What your number means
Folate	ng/ml	Also known as B9. Plays a role in the growth and repair, as well as the production, of healthy red blood cells.	Low levels may contribute to anaemia and lead to decreased energy.
Thyroid Function TSH, T4, T3	TSH: mlU/L T3 and T4: pmol/L	The thyroid gland produces hormones that help to regulate the body's metabolism.	When thyroid hormones are too high or too low, they can impact how every cell in the body functions.
Complete blood count	Various units	Provides a detailed anlaysis of different components of your blood by measuring the number, size and composition of your various blood cells, including red blood cells, white blood cells and platelets.	When the size or composition of the various blood cells are outside of normal ranges they can signal conditions, such as anaemia or signs of an infection.

Advanced metabolic health blood tests can also be obtained privately

Private labs can run more advanced blood tests to assess a further range of markers that can indicate your risk factor for suffering metabolic health issues early. For example fasting insulin is a vital and valuable marker that provides an early warning sign if your energy system is faltering.

Some direct-to-consumer private lab testing companies:
— **Medichecks** *medichecks.com*
— **Thriva** *thriva.co*
— **Monitor my health** *monitormyhealth.org.uk*
— **One Day Tests** *onedaytests.com*

Alternately, you can go direct to a registered nutritionist or healthcare provider to build a bespoke testing package that includes more superior markers to evaluate risk factors, as well as help you to identify any low nutrient levels.

Other tests you can do at home
— **Blood pressure**
— **Body composition:** you can purchase analyser scales, a tool that evaluates body composition. There are many scales on the market now that can measure more than just weight; they can tell you your muscle mass and fat mass percentage. They may not be 100 per cent accurate but provide a baseline to work with and can be used to track progress over time.
— **Waist circumference**

Continuous glucose monitor (CGM)
For more information on the benefits of purchasing one for a two-week trial, see page 83.
— **Lingo** *hellolingo.com*

Recipes

*I have shared with you a few of the recipes I rely on weekly.
I consider them to be staple dishes that help maintain
stable energy. They are simple, quick and a few of them
you can make in bulk to eat across the week.*

Green protein smoothie guide

Protein smoothies are a great way to increase nutrient
density and eat functional foods in a convenient way.
It is important to balance the smoothie appropriately to
support metabolic health. Here is a framework of what
to include in your smoothie:

— **Protein:** 1–2 scoops of a good-quality protein powder
  (or a few tablespoons of Greek yoghurt/soy yoghurt/
  silken tofu)

— **Micronutrients:** 1–2 handfuls of leafy green vegetables,
  for example, spinach or kale

— **Flavour/polyphenol:** 1 handful of berries

— **Fibre:** 1–2 tablespoons of chia seeds or flaxseed

— **Liquid:** milk of your choice

— **Optional extras to add creaminess:** ½ avocado,
  1–2 tablespoons of nut butter or yoghurt

— **Flavour enhancers:** cocoa powder (unsweetened),
  ground cinnamon, matcha

A note on protein powders

A good-quality protein powder should contain minimal, high-quality ingredients, without artificial additives, fillers or sweeteners. Look for a protein powder that meets the following criteria:

— **Protein source:** pure, high-quality sources like grass-fed whey or plant-based proteins like pea, hemp or brown rice.

— **Minimal ingredients:** the ingredients list should have no more than 5–6 items.

— **Avoid the following artificial sweeteners:** aspartame, sucralose, saccharin or acesulfame potassium.

— **Natural sweeteners:** if the powder contains a sweetener look for natural options like stevia, monk fruit, or organic coconut sugar in small amounts.

— **No artificial flavours or colours:** opt for unflavoured powders or those with natural flavours and spices, herbs and fruit powders.

— **Third-party tested:** choose a protein powder that has been third-party tested for purity, potency and safety. Check the brand's website or contact the manufactuer.

Grain-free porridge with natural yoghurt

A fibre-rich meal that is a good alternative to porridge and a great way to start the day.

Serves 2
—

250–300ml full-fat coconut milk or unsweetened almond milk with no added sugars or oil
3 tbsp chia seeds
2 tbsp unsweetened coconut flakes
2 tbsp ground flaxseed
2 tbsp hemp seed hearts
2 tbsp ground almonds or coconut flour
1 tsp ground cinnamon
1 tsp raw honey (optional)
1 scoop of collagen powder or protein powder (optional)
2 handfuls of berries, to serve
Greek or coconut yoghurt, to serve

Heat the milk in a small pan over a medium heat until hot but not boiling.

Turn the heat off then stir in the chia seeds, coconut flakes, flaxseed, hemp seed hearts, almond or coconut flour, cinnamon and honey, if using.

Stir for about a minute until the porridge has thickened, then stir in the collagen powder or protein powder, if using. Add a handful of berries to each portion and serve with yoghurt.

Chia seed overnight oats with blueberries

A great alternative to porridge, packed with omega-3 fat, fibre and polyphenols.

Serves 1
—

20g oats (jumbo or steel-cut)
2 tbsp chia seeds
200–240ml unsweetened plant-based milk
with no added oils
a handful of berries
2 tbsp yoghurt (coconut yoghurt or full-fat
Greek yoghurt)
1 tbsp nut butter (optional)
2 tsp cocoa nibs (optional)
unsweetened shredded coconut (optional)
1 scoop of protein powder or collagen powder
(optional)

Mix the ingredients together in a bowl, place in a sealed jar and leave overnight, adding any optional extras.

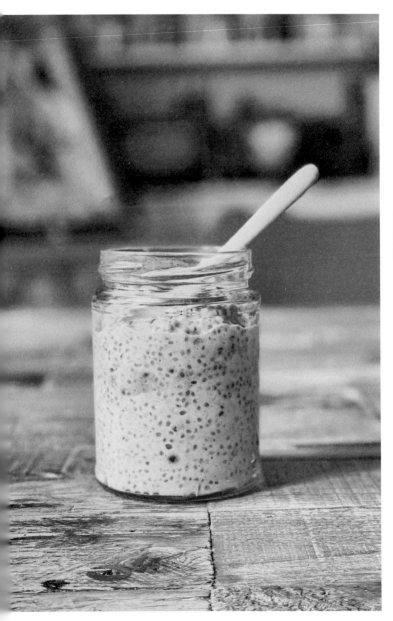

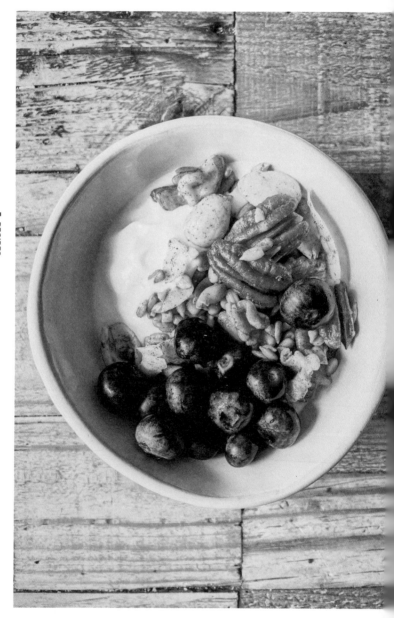

Nut and seed granola

I have been making granola for years now—they are packed with fibre and healthy fats. I make one in bulk once a week for my family, adding the cacao powder and a few cups of oats for my daughter. Feel free to adjust the nuts and seeds. Serve with yoghurt and berries.

Makes about 10 servings
—

130g almonds
120g sunflower seeds or pumpkin seeds (or both)
50g walnuts
50g pecans
1–2 tsp ground cinnamon
20g coconut oil
a pinch of salt
1 tbsp raw cacao powder (optional)
25g unsweetened shredded coconut
50g hemp seed hearts

Preheat the oven to 180°C fan (350°F). Line a baking sheet with parchment paper.

In a large bowl, mix together the almonds, sunflower seeds, walnuts, pecans, cinnamon, coconut oil, salt, and cacao powder if using. Spread out on the baking sheet.

Bake the granola for 8 minutes, stirring halfway. Be sure to watch it closely so that it does not burn.

Remove from the oven and pour into a large bowl. Add the shredded coconut and hemp seeds and mix well.

Allow to cool before serving. Keep for up to a week in an airtight container.

Flaxseed wraps

I know that many people can often miss bread and wraps. This is my go-to wrap — high in fibre, so simple to make and takes no time at all. Serve with the rainbow salad opposite and a protein source.

Serves 1

—

2 tbsp ground flaxseed
¼ tsp any dried herb or spice you like
(I love oregano or paprika)
¼ tsp baking powder
1 large egg
1 tbsp water
1 garlic clove, crushed or chopped
1–2 tsp coconut oil
sea salt and black pepper

In a small bowl mix together the flaxseed, dried herb or spice and baking powder.

In another small bowl whisk the egg, water and garlic, season with salt and pepper, then add to the flaxseed mix to make a batter.

Heat the coconut oil in a pan, pour in the batter and spread evenly. Heat until cooked through — for about 30 seconds to 1 minute, until no longer moist. Flip over and cook for another 30 seconds.

Rainbow coleslaw salad

An antioxidant, polyphenol-rich salad. Make it in bulk and serve with your main meals. Your gut will love you! Serve with beans, organic tofu, eggs and top with pecans and hazelnuts. You can store the coleslaw in an airtight container in the fridge for 4–5 days.

Serves 4–6 as a side

—

½ red or white cabbage (I love to mix both),
    thinly sliced
1 small red onion, finely chopped
1 orange or yellow pepper (or ½ of both), thinly sliced
2 carrots, thinly sliced
¼ cucumber, diced
a large handful of coriander or flat-leaf parsley,
    roughly chopped
1–2 tbsp extra virgin olive oil
1 tbsp raw apple cider vinegar
1 red chilli, chopped (optional)
seeds from ½–1 pomegranate
capers (optional)
sea salt and black pepper

Mix all the ingredients in a large bowl, adding capers and seasoning to your taste.

I really enjoy this salad using a tahini dressing — 1–2 tbsp tahini, 1–2 tbsp water, ½ lemon freshly squeezed, 1 tsp Dijon mustard, 1 clove of chopped or crushed garlic, salt and pepper to taste — mix all the ingredients in a bowl until combined and add to the salad ingredients.

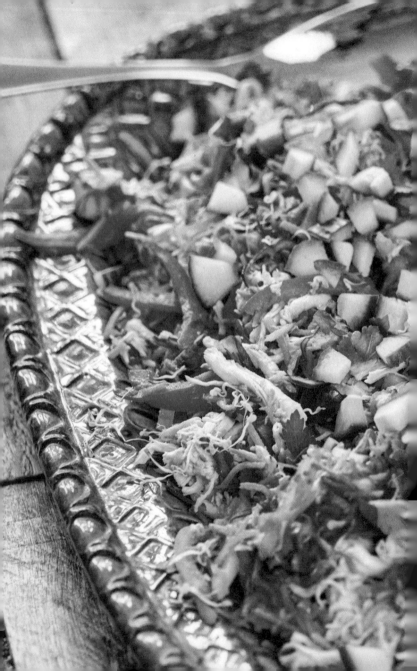

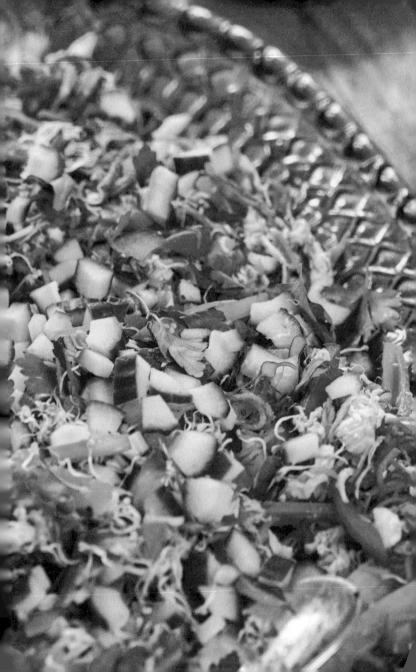

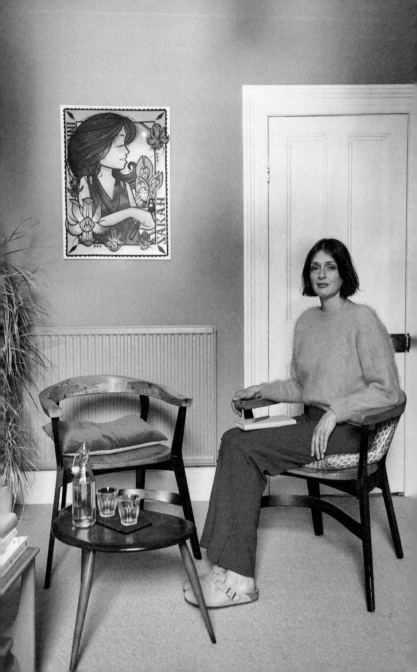

About the author

Sarah is a registered nutritional therapist with a private practice in Bristol, England, specialising in metabolic health, stress management and sustaining energy levels. Her mission is to help people protect their vitality, mitigate potential health risk factors and build resilience. She does this through bespoke client work, talks and workshops.

Sarah's determination was sparked at the age of 12 when she was diagnosed with severe dyslexia. Fuelled by a desire to overcome challenges and succeed, she earned a first-class distinction degree in Marketing, just a decade after learning to read and write. She went on to have a successful 15-year career in marketing, managing accounts for major clients like Diageo and Unilever.

After experiencing burnout, Sarah became fascinated by the effects of lifestyle on the body, mind and soul. This led her to become certified by the world-renowned College of Naturopathic Medicine, and become a member of the Institute for Functional Medicine with AFMCP certification.

Sarah is a member of BANT (British Association for Applied Nutrition and Nutritional Therapy), which is the professional body for nutritional therapists. She is also registered with the CNHC (Complementary and Natural Healthcare Council), the regulatory body for complementary health.

You can connect with Sarah via her website: *sarahbaylissnutrition.co.uk* or via social media *@sarahbayliss_nutrition*

Thanks

My sincere thanks to...

My dad, my biggest champion. Through all the ups and downs, you've pushed me, believed in me, and fought my corner. Thank you for your constant encouragement and those tough talks that kept me going when I needed them most.

To my courageous mum, you've accomplished incredible things and shown me that anything is truly possible. Thank you for inspiring me to take those leaps of faith.

Chris, my wonderful husband, and rock since the day we met. That day is still vivid in my mind; you surprised me then and continue to do so every day. I'm deeply grateful for your belief in me, even when I doubt myself.

To my little one, you're teaching me so much about myself, and life. Being your mum is the greatest adventure, and I'm thankful for every moment.

To the amazing people who have shaped my journey in writing this book:

A heartfelt thank you to Mark Shayler, for recognising the potential in my work, believing in me, and being the catalyst behind this book.

To the wonderful Mike Coulter, who trusted my advice and has since wholeheartedly supported and encouraged me with great enthusiasm. A huge thank you too, for introducing me to The DO Lectures.

To David and Clare Hieatt for inviting me to speak at The DO Lectures, seeing something in me and my story, and for helping me.

To David Scotland, your guidance and coaching has been invaluable in helping me find the confidence and strength to tell my story.

To my publisher Miranda West and my editor, Imogen Fortes, thank you for recognising value in my words and believing they were worth sharing.

To Christian Banfield, your photography is simply stunning, and your brand guidance has been invaluable. Thank you!

To all my clients, thank you for entrusting me with your health and wellbeing.

Finally, to you reading this right now, thank you for your time. It means more than you know.

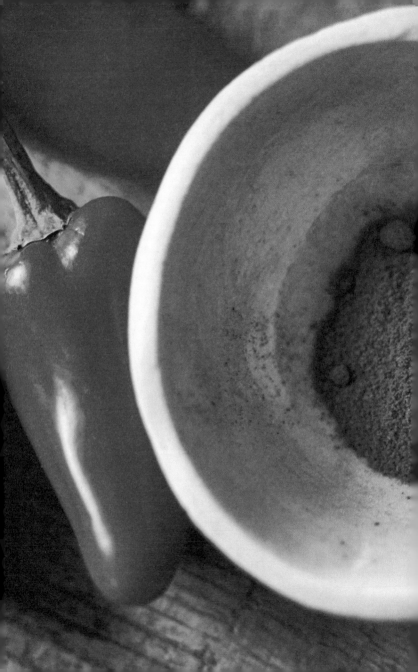

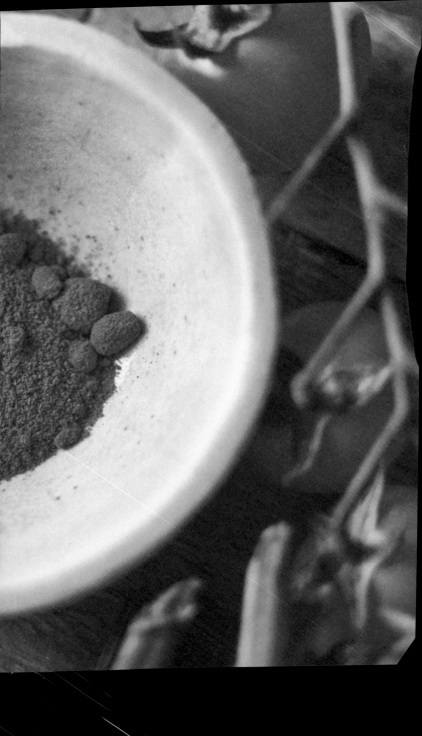

Books in the series

Available in print, digital and audio formats from booksellers or via our
website: **thedobook.co**. To hear about events and forthcoming titles,
find us on social media **@dobookco**, or subscribe to our newsletter.